Bernadette Ward

CAM, An Irish Solution to a Global Question?

To my lovely
Yas,
Much love

Mum

Bernadette

x/x/

Bernadette Ward

CAM, An Irish Solution to a Global Question?

Analysis of the Complementary and Alternative Medicine Sector

LAP LAMBERT Academic Publishing

Impressum / Imprint
Bibliografische Information der Deutschen Nationalbibliothek: Die Deutsche Nationalbibliothek verzeichnet diese Publikation in der Deutschen Nationalbibliografie; detaillierte bibliografische Daten sind im Internet über http://dnb.d-nb.de abrufbar.
Alle in diesem Buch genannten Marken und Produktnamen unterliegen warenzeichen-, marken- oder patentrechtlichem Schutz bzw. sind Warenzeichen oder eingetragene Warenzeichen der jeweiligen Inhaber. Die Wiedergabe von Marken, Produktnamen, Gebrauchsnamen, Handelsnamen, Warenbezeichnungen u.s.w. in diesem Werk berechtigt auch ohne besondere Kennzeichnung nicht zu der Annahme, dass solche Namen im Sinne der Warenzeichen- und Markenschutzgesetzgebung als frei zu betrachten wären und daher von jedermann benutzt werden dürften.

Bibliographic information published by the Deutsche Nationalbibliothek: The Deutsche Nationalbibliothek lists this publication in the Deutsche Nationalbibliografie; detailed bibliographic data are available in the Internet at http://dnb.d-nb.de.
Any brand names and product names mentioned in this book are subject to trademark, brand or patent protection and are trademarks or registered trademarks of their respective holders. The use of brand names, product names, common names, trade names, product descriptions etc. even without a particular marking in this work is in no way to be construed to mean that such names may be regarded as unrestricted in respect of trademark and brand protection legislation and could thus be used by anyone.

Coverbild / Cover image: www.ingimage.com

Verlag / Publisher:
LAP LAMBERT Academic Publishing
ist ein Imprint der / is a trademark of
OmniScriptum GmbH & Co. KG
Heinrich-Böcking-Str. 6-8, 66121 Saarbrücken, Deutschland / Germany
Email: info@lap-publishing.com

Herstellung: siehe letzte Seite /
Printed at: see last page
ISBN: 978-3-659-30230-5

Zugl. / Approved by: Dublin, Ireland, Dublin City University, Dissertation 2014

Acknowledgements

Firstly I would like to all of the CAM participants, both national and international, who gave their time to either complete the questionnaires or to take part in the in depth interviews, which helped me to form this study, and write this manuscript.

I would like to express my gratitude to Dr. Joe O Hara for his help and encouragement.

I would also like to thank Dr. Gerry McNamara who encouraged my participation in the Doctorate programme, from the beginning.

Finally, I would like to thank my family, Mark, for his help and encouragement, Shannon and Yasmin for encouraging and supporting me, and not least Finn and Zoe, whose learning journey is just beginning.

Contents

List of Tables

List of Figures

Glossary of Acronyms

CAM	Complementary and Alternative Medicine
DOHC	Department for Health and Children
ECTS	European Credit Transfer System
EU	European Union
EFQ	European Quality Framework
FETAC	Further Education and Training Awards Council
HEI	Higher Education Ireland
HETAC	Higher Education and Training Awards Council
IPA	Irish Public Administration
IUQB	Irish University Qualifications Board
NFQ	National Frameworks of Qualifications
NQAI	National Qualifications Authority Ireland
NWG	National Working Group
QA	Quality Assurance
OECD	Organisation of Economic and Cultural Development
QQI	Quality and Qualifications Ireland
RDS	Royal Dublin Society
SMCI	SMCI Consultants Limited
TQM	Total Quality Management
TM	Traditional Medicine
TNA	Training Needs Analysis
UNESCO	United Nations Educational Scientific and Cultural Organisation.

Chapter 1 Overview

1.1 Introduction

CAM (Complementary and Alternative Medicines) or natural healing has been part of public healthcare choices in Ireland from early monastic times, when cures were sought and used for a range of ailments. Natural healing predates biomedicine and has remained a popular choice down through the ages, to current times. Often described as *"alternative"* to the more accepted, scientific biomedical systems used by most countries for their healthcare systems. The World Health Organisation in their publication on General Guidelines for Methodologies for Research and Evaluation of Traditional Medicine Research have observed that the terms used describing native, traditional medicines vary from country to country.

> *"The terms complementary/alternative/non-conventional medicine are used interchangeably with traditional medicine in some countries" WHO (2000 Pg.1).*

More recently defined by the natural and holistic healthcare sectors as Complementary Medicine, the term CAM is now widely used to describe a range of ancient and modern healing practices, which fall outside of the officially accepted healthcare systems in Ireland and other countries. Ibid

> *"The term complementary and alternative medicine is used in some countries to refer to a broad set of health care practices that are not part of the country's own tradition and are not integrated into the dominant health care system" WHO (2000 Pg.. 1)*

Despite the dominance of biomedicine, many countries acknowledge their traditional healing roots. Both the EU and the WHO have sought to map, record and make recommendations for the protection and recognition of non-dominant traditional medicines. WHO (2005).

The study on which this book is based seeks to examine the CAM community in Ireland, explore how learning is delivered and practitioners are created. It seeks to explore public demand for treatments and the provision of learning for courses in complementary therapies, examining if there is any oversight in terms of quality of learning, or regulation of practice in Ireland. It further seeks to identify and define the needs of this community in terms of their continued survival and growth within the broader healthcare sector in Ireland and makes some comparisons to other countries with similar population demands, healthcare systems and community structures. Through the examination of the historical background of CAM in Ireland and the current status, the study seeks to identify gaps in terms of what this community needs.

1.1 1 Chapter Outlines

Chapter One outlines the study rationale and objectives, detailing research questions and aspects of the study the research questions seek to answer. It discusses the current status of learning and practice in Ireland which underpins the study rationale. The chapter outlines how the CAM community was shaped within the historical background of Ireland of thirty years ago, when this community first began to emerge. It discusses how Ireland`s membership and active participation in international organisations such as the EU, OECD helped shape Irish government policy on adult and lifelong learning. The CAM sector as a significant provider of lifelong learning is discussed in this chapter in relation to second chance education for adult learners, as most CAM learners are mature students seeking further or higher education.

Chapter Two outlines the key literature selected for relevance to the research questions and examines the literature in relation to several aspects of the study objectives. Literature on public demand and regulation of complementary therapies considered to be fundamental to the study is explored and demonstrates a demand for CAM treatments, relevant to the training of therapists to provide treatments. Available material on the regulation of CAM therapies in

Ireland including previous DOHC initiatives is examined and discussed, so as to provide a background to the study on the current status of this sector. This relates to a review of publications on academic validation and professional accreditation of CAM courses in Ireland and an examination of available literature on obstacles to recognition of complementary therapies. This latter material was examined in relation to a lack of progress and reported resistance to the regulation of this sector, both in Ireland and elsewhere. Adult and Higher education in Ireland and how it is provided and graded in relation to qualifications is explored by examining the National Framework of Qualifications which is mapped within this chapter. Literature on civil rights and the consumers right to choose is explored and discussed, as it is relevant to the consumer's right to choose a CAM treatment as a healthcare option. Finally relevant literature on quality assurance, its evolution in Ireland within the education system and in educational reform in both adult and higher education in Ireland and the EU is discussed and reviewed.

In Chapter Three the methodological paradigm and the thinking which guided the study is described. It discusses the rationale as to why a post positivist mixed methodology was used in both data collection and data analysis and how the study was planned within that framework. The study focus of a community's needs analysis which guided the investigation is described and it outlines and discusses the research tools and sequencing used in order to identify the concerns and needs of this sector. The rationale behind the research sample both in terms of the questionnaire and the interview elements of the study was discussed. Finally study triangulation in the use of mixed methods to explore the research questions and generalisation of the study to the wider CAM community is discussed.

Chapter Four discusses data collection and the thought process and sequencing used in the designing and planning of both the online questionnaire, and the stakeholder interviews which followed. The online questionnaire was designed to include both quantitative and qualitative elements in the form of closed questions to survey information and comment text boxes used to provide respondent comments. It describes sample recruitment for both the questionnaire and the stakeholder interviews. This chapter discusses the designing of guide questions for the semi-structured stakeholder interviews, the interview process and conditions. It discusses interview participants, how they were recruited and the interviews arranged. Finally it describes the recording and the transcription of the interviews, the organisation and preparation of transcripts for analysis within the methods chosen for the study.

Chapter Five begins by outlining the analysis of both the quantitative and qualitative data derived from the study. It describes the use of survey software to analyse the quantitative data and the thematic analysis methodology for the analysis of the qualitative data. The chapter details the study results and findings from both the quantitative and qualitative data sources. It outlines and discusses the themes which emerged from the raw data and maps the dominant themes and concepts of both methodologies in a discussion of the findings and how they relate to the research questions. Each emerging theme is identified and discussed in relation to the study focused needs analysis of the CAM community, in terms of both the quantitative and qualitative data findings. It discussed the use of the mixed methods in data gathering and analysis as a complementary and collaborative exercise and described how both the quantitative and qualitative data was integrated in the findings of the study in order to answer the research questions.

Chapter Six discusses the findings of both the quantitative and qualitative data and the implications of the findings for the CAM community. It describes the concerns, priorities and needs of the community which emerged from the data collected in both datasets. Within this chapter the impact of the current situation on the CAM community is discussed and data that emerged from the study relating to the research questions is described. It discussed the comparisons to the CAM community in the UK and internationally in terms of recognition and public access to therapies. This chapter outlines the needs of this community which emerged from the data, and recommendations on how the sector could be improved, and the changes that could be made which could strengthen the CAM sector as a whole Finally, it outlines the limitations of this research and makes recommendations for further research.

1.1.2 Key Research Questions

The following questions addressed in order to analyse the CAM sector in Ireland and explore its past and present status and current concerns. The study examines the Irish CAM community in terms of recognition, regulation and status of the sector. It also examines the provision of education and training of therapists and the status of professional practice of CAM therapies in Ireland. Finally it explores what are the current issues and concerns that impact on the community and what their priorities and needs are for the future. The key research questions addressed therefore are

- Who are the main Irish CAM stakeholders and what are their roles and experiences?
- Does the lack of recognition and regulation impact on CAM Training and Practice?
- What - if any quality -oversight is there for training and practice in the CAM sector?
- Has it been necessary for CAM Learning Providers to go outside of Ireland to achieve academic validation?
- What are the current issues, concerns and needs of the CAM sector?

1.2 Study Background, Rationale and Objectives

The study investigates aspects of complementary and alternative medicine education, training and practice in Ireland relevant to the research questions. As a comparative analysis it also investigates training and practice in the UK and other countries where conditions are similar, Ward (2009). The topic was chosen as there is a paucity of research from within the field of CAM education and training in Ireland, and there remains a gap in the existing literature within this sector. What limited research carried out has been from outside of the sector from the wider healthcare communities. An extensive literature review showed that this subject had not been addressed in previous studies.

The CAM sector is a broadly based community of mature adults who can be seen as taking on the roles of both learners and practitioners. In many cases students undertaking education and training in a CAM therapy are returning to education and characteristically fit into the category of lifelong learning. They deliberately choose complementary therapies to either add to existing skills or to acquire a new skill or competency which will improve their employment opportunities. In the researcher's experience from working in the community that CAM students, express a long term interest and motivation to study in one or more therapies. Provision of education and training across the complementary therapy sector meets a steady and consistent public demand for therapists in a variety of disciplines, and establishes a significant private education sector, McDonagh, Devine & Baxter (2007).

There is a strong demand within Ireland, the UK and the English speaking world for CAM treatments of one type or another, CAMbrella (2012), This is reflected in a similar steady and constant demand reported across the EU and documented in relevant literature which forms part of this study's Literature Review, Ernst & White (2000), WHO (2005), DOHC (2002), DOHC (2005). Despite consumer demonstrations of choice in sourcing and paying for treatments, the CAM sector within the EU and most of the English speaking world remains unregulated and unsupported by successive governments, Budd & Mills (2000 Pg. 8).

There are no national registers of adequately trained and regulated CAM therapists and citizens within Ireland and the EU are left to their own devices to search for competent and safe practitioners, CAMbrella(2012).

Patients will go to great lengths to source a particular treatment, as there are no government registers and will make their own judgements and evaluations on the treatments.

> *"Patients are informed consumers and not naive participants, as they research practitioners as best they can by "word of mouth" before consulting and judge their continuation of treatments by the results. They will continue to seek and pay for treatments they find to be effective for their conditions even if the situation remains the same", Ward (2009 Pg.74).*

The lack of guidance and recommendations on possible structures or frameworks in which complementary and alternative medicine could be acknowledged and recognised both in terms of training, regulation and practice is noted in the CAMbrella Report to the EU (2012). There is no evidence that this report has been acted on or has resulted in any further action or progression of the status of CAM within the EU and its member states. Arguably demands of inclusion and equity, require EU policy makers and therefore its member states to address these issues, but this does not seem to be the case and indeed EU states actively discriminate against complementary and alternative medicine, in terms or training, regulation and practice. It could be argued that governmental policy makers have not yet found a relevant process with which to regulate CAM training and practice, and the lack of scientific evidence of effect for some of the therapies is one of the reasons often used by government agencies as to why they have difficulties in agreeing regulation policy. There is no doubt that governments, including the Irish government are uncertain as to how to categorise this sector and how to find a place for them within national policy, DOHC (2005), Lords Report (2002), Budd & Mills (2000).

19

Perhaps one of the strongest arguments to be made with regards to the need for regulation in the CAM sector is that of public safety. Members of the public seeking out treatments cannot consult practitioner registers or seek official guidance, so they make their own judgements to seek out a range of therapeutic or healthcare treatments, some of which are invasive, without any government oversight. Dismissal of CAM treatments by doctors and the wider healthcare professions as "quackery" is not an effective argument in attempting to steer patients away from CAM treatments. Anecdotal evidence of good effects from one or other treatments within the population is enough to motivate patients to seek out therapists.

> "Limitation of treatment options available to patients does not work. They want access to a treatment which works for them and it is essential this access be provided from a controlled safe source. If it is not available from a safe source they will continue to seek it anyway", Ward (2009 Pg. 65).

If the response to enquiries to their doctors is always negative, they will just stop reporting their experiences to their GPs. They want to be able to choose their own healthcare options, alongside their medical treatments, as in Ireland, the majority of people pay for both medical and complementary medical treatments, Budd & Mills (2000).

> "Patients need freedom of choice and the right to access an acknowledged safe source of practitioners, preferably within the conventional healthcare structures. Ward (2009 Pg. 54).

1.2.1 Statement of Interest

As a researcher, my interest in this area emerged from more than twenty five years of active involvement in Acupuncture and Chinese Medicine training and practice in Ireland. My involvement in the

CAM sector was focused on education and training of therapists and the establishment of professional associations to provide for their registration. I have been active within and head a private CAM learning provider delivering skills based training to adult learners and have direct experience of working within the sector. In this role, I have worked on a process of quality assurance design and approval with HETAC, NQAI and more recently QQI in efforts to achieve academic validation for a CAM training programme. As part of my academic studies, I completed a Master of Science degree in Traditional Chinese Medicine in London's Middlesex University, for which I received an academic award. My research for the taught Masters programme was a two centre study in both Dublin and London and focused on how the lack of regulation of Complementary Therapists impacts on the clinical relationship from both the practitioner and patient point of view. The current study which is the focus of this publication is a continuation of a body of work from within the CAM sector to explore CAM sector needs. It has a focus on training and professional practice, and explores acknowledgement and recognition of student learning within the CAM community in Ireland and elsewhere. On completion of this study and following four years of a taught Doctoral programme in Dublin City University, I graduated with a Doctor of Education award, of which this research formed part of my course work. Research subjectivity and bias is addressed in Chapter Three of this publication.

1.3 CAM History and Context

Within the world of Complementary and Alternative Medicine, organised education and training courses in Ireland did not begin to appear until the early eighties. Advertisements for single informal courses in Reflexology, Acupressure, and Transcendental Meditation began appearing in national and local newspapers canvassing for students. Typically these were organised by therapists who had learned their skills outside of Ireland and who now were offering training in therapies they themselves had learned. Courses were offered to adult learners on a part time, fee paying basis. In several cases individual therapists offered training courses without any organisational or institutional structures in place. Courses were delivered in a variety of venues, ranging from hotel meeting rooms, to classrooms rented on weekends and evenings in educational institutions. They formed a variation of theory and skills demonstration and practice and graduates were certified as therapists by the providers in whatever discipline they were being taught.

The social context in which these courses began to be offered was one of emerging public demand for healthcare options other than those offered by their doctors and hospitals. It was not an either/or situation as patients typically attended their doctors as well as a complementary therapist.

> *Patients do consult their GPs first for their conditions and only when they find they cannot get effective treatment or medication with unacceptable side effects do they consult a practitioner ",Ward (2009 Pg.74).*

The Irish have a tradition of seeking natural healthcare treatments, such as, bone setters, faith healers, seventh sons of seventh sons, those who were perceived to have a "gift" of healing. From the early eighties annual alternative health conferences began to be organised for the public to attend in the main cities, such as the Mind Body Spirit seminars which were organised in large exhibition places such as the Mansion House and the RDS in Dublin. Educational talks were given to the public and members of the public could try or test a variety of treatments at these events. These exhibitions or seminars also took place in other main cities, and across the UK with similar themes and all were equally well attended. There were at the time responding to an emerging public demand for information on complementary therapies and were primarily used to deliver public information and for some to canvass for students of the various therapies being demonstrated.

Table 1.1 outlines the main CAM therapies most active and popular, some from the early eighties, who remain in demand both in terms of training and practice to the current day. There are additionally a variety of other therapies not included in this table, they have not been excluded for any particular reason other than the focus of this study is the most commonly known therapies and those defined by the Department of Health and Children Report on the Regulation of Complementary Therapists (DOHC 2005).

Public information on training and treatment was in the early days provided in leaflets and brochures, and in the intervening years some therapies enjoyed a steady growth in popularity. Training Programmes in Acupuncture, Homoeopathy, Herbalism, Reflexology and Massage began to be advertised in Ireland and CAM training courses became a common element of adult learning in Ireland over the past thirty years. Many graduates of a diversity of CAM programmes began to offer their services to the public, outlining the benefits of their treatments. Therapists began registering with the professional associations and became part of what has now become an active CAM community. Today most CAM professional associations have public information websites furnishing details of their organisations, treatments and in many cases lists of their professional members. The following table outlines the most active CAM therapies in Ireland.

Therapy	Source of training	Courses available from	Reference
Acupuncture	Irish courses	Circa 1985	www.afpa.ie www.tcmci.ie
Chiropractic	Not taught in Ireland	Circa 1983	
Chinese Herbalism	Irish courses	Circa 1992	www.achi.ie www.irchm.ie
Herbalism (Western)	Irish Courses	Circa 1999	www.ihr.ie
Homoeopathy	Irish Courses	Circa 1990	www.ishom.ie
Iridology	Irish Courses	Circa 1999	www.herbeire.ie
Massage (various)	Irish Courses	Circa 1980	www.ficta.ie
Osteopathy	Practiced but not taught in Ireland	Circa 1990	www.osteopathy.ie
Reflexology	Irish Courses	Circa 1983	www.reflexology.ie
Reiki	Irish Courses	Circa 1995	www.reikifederation.ie
Federation of CAM Therapies(various)	Irish Courses	Circa 2003	www.ficta.ie

Table 1.1: CAM Therapies in Ireland
*Dates are approximate and based on available information on the various therapies.

1.4 CAM and the Irish Adult Education System

The Irish CAM education sector has never been analysed as by its nature it has fallen outside of the traditional educational structures. Just as the public will seek out a complementary medical treatment, those interested, will also seek out training in a CAM therapy. It is also the direct experience of the researcher that those interested in training in a complementary therapy will look for competence in that therapy though government oversight is not a first priority. Indeed there is often an acknowledgement by potential students that there may not be government recognition of their CAM qualification. Perhaps for this reason learning providers have not typically focused on government recognition in the promotion of their programmes to potential students.

Nevertheless, it is arguable that the learning journey which many adults begin when they study one complementary therapy, and often go on to study another should in an ideal world be acknowledged and recognised by the relevant government agencies. It could be argued that Ireland's membership of international organisations such as the EU and the OECD who have developed policies on recognition of all learning could influence the Irish government policy with regard to the recognition of learning within the CAM sector.

1.4.1 The OECD, Ireland and Recognition of Adult Learning

The OECD (Organisation for Economic Co-operation and Development) was established in 1948 under a US financed initiative to promote national inter dependency, following the devastation of the 2nd world war. The initiative developed on a global scale, with an international membership of 34 countries.

> *"Today, 34 OECD member countries worldwide regularly turn to one another to identify problems, discuss and analyse them, and promote policies to solve them" OECD website homepage (2014).*

It provides a forum for member countries to cooperate on social, economic and environmental issues and can help national policy makers solve problems.

> *"The Organisation provides a setting where governments can compare policy experiences, seek answers to common problems, identify good practice and work to co-ordinate domestic and international policies", Ibid.*

The European Commission works closely with the OECD as most countries are members of both organisational structures as is Ireland. Progress and enlightenment is a stated core policy of the OECD for its member national populations, and in 1996 member Education Ministers agreed to develop strategies for lifelong learning to be shared across its member populations. In a paper which emerged from the OECD Education Directorate in 2007 a definition of lifelong learning was agreed and defined. This was intended to address the different terms and perceptions of learning in all its forms. They viewed economic growth and progress within member countries to be directly linked to adult learning within its populations, in whatever form that took. The definition of all forms of learning was a first step in acknowledgement and recognition of all adult learning.

"The concept of "from cradle to grave" includes formal, non-formal, and informal learning. It is an approach whose importance may now be clearer than ever and non-formal and informal learning outcomes are viewed as having significant value. Policy-makers in many OECD countries, and beyond, are therefore trying to develop strategies to use all the skills, knowledge and competences – wherever they come from – individuals may have at a time when countries are striving to reap the benefits of economic growth, global competitiveness and population development", OECD (2007).

They decided in their definition of learning to use two analytic descriptions, Learning Outcomes and Intentionality, or Deliberate learning. This was an acknowledgement of the variety of learning approaches across member states designed for adult learners. In their agreement of these definitions OECD members took the position that all learning has value and should be acknowledged and recognised both nationally and internationally.

The following table outlines the OECD definitions of those three types of learning.

Formal Learning	They may learn during courses or during training session in the workplace. The activity is designed as having learning objectives and individuals attend with the explicit goal of acquiring skills, knowledge or competence.
Non-Formal Learning	They may learn during work or leisure activities that do not have learning objectives but individuals are aware they are learning; this is non-formal learning. Individuals observe or do things with the intention of becoming more skilled, more knowledgeable and/or more competent
Informal Learning	They may learn during activities with learning objectives but they learn beyond the learning objectives; this is semi-

	formal learning. This is a new term that is proposed here. Individuals have the intention of learning about something and, without knowing it, learn also about something else; and they may learn in activities without learning objectives and without knowing they are learning.

Table 1.2:   OECD Definitions of learning (2005 Pg. 5).

They focused on acknowledgement, and recognition of learning which would mean certification of learning, in whatever form that would take, within member states national institutions and societies. The OECD took the view that learning should be acknowledged as having taken place and could be recognised socially with the awarding of certification for formal learning, Werquin (2008 Pg. 144).

They advocated that *"all learning had value and most of it deserves to be made visible and recognised"* They stated that all individuals engaging in deliberate intentional learning with learning outcomes should be recognised by their national institutions and that they should be acknowledged with certification.

Commenting on this Werquin writing about lifelong learning in Europe, argued

> "The recognition of non-formal and informal learning mechanically improves the qualification distribution of the population (and not only the young generations) with little additional burden on the formal education and training system", Ibid (Pg. 145).

Several countries have no system of recognition or of coding non-formal or informal learning within national qualification frameworks. The OECD, post 2007, has made it a priority to inform and encourage member nations to develop a system of recognition for all types of learning, in order to address the social and economic needs of the future. Werquin writes

> "The recognition of non-formal and informal learning is an important means for making the 'lifelong learning for all' agenda a reality for all and, subsequently, for reshaping learning to better match the needs of the 21st century knowledge economies and open societies", Ibid.

CAM training fits into the lifelong learning model as typically adult learners take part in formal and non- formal training, and a government policy to acknowledge all learning would benefit CAM learners, and provide social recognition for their learning effort.

1.4.2 Ireland and the OECD

Ireland became a full member of the OECD in 1961, and has been an active participant within this forum. A search of the OECD website, member state pages, produces a number of academic papers published by Irish academics relating to current forum issues illustrating Ireland's contribution to OECD initiatives and activities.

Ireland actively participated in the OECD initiative on recognition of all types of adult learning. This included active participation in a 2006/07 OECD activity, which resulted in the publication of a report on the recognition of all learning. This report was drafted by the Irish qualifications and higher education agencies, NQAI and HETAC and demonstrates Ireland`s commitment to recognition of lifelong learning.

Previously in 2005 Ireland took part in an OECD pilot project to test best practice on the recognition of non-formal and informal learning initially focusing on providers of education and training in the Further Education sector.

> *"Ireland introduced a pilot project with nine learning providers, help from the Further Education and Training Award Council (FETAC), and some 50 participants. The aim is simultaneously to undertake the recognition of non-formal and informal learning outcomes with a small group of providers, to identify good practice and problems, and to exchange experience as regards what works well", OECD (2007 Pg. 33).*

This was one of the initiatives relating to OECD policy of recognition of adult and lifelong learning. The OECD country report for Ireland was intended to document Ireland`s status with regard to recognition of prior learning, both informal and non-formal by Irish institutions. Irish government policy is documented as having a position of acknowledgement and recognition of non-formal and informal learning in line with both OECD and EU concepts of progress, inclusion and equality. This position did not transfer into an acknowledgement of learning undertaken by the many adult learners undertaking CAM training. As providers of learning to adult learners the complementary and alternative medicine sector was not included in the OECD pilot study on acknowledgement of all types of learning or of government agency policy initiatives. Although there is no information available as to why this sector was not included, it could be argued that as there was no government policy with regard to this sector as a whole, inclusion in government initiatives, without recognition of the sector may have presented difficulties for FETAC.

1.4.3 Ireland and EU Policy on Lifelong Learning

Ireland, as an active member state of the European Union has fully participated in European educational goals and policies, since the beginning of the EU and EEC, despite historical national conservatism and traditions. Wolfgang Horner and Hans Dorbert, writing on the Education Systems of Europe state that education systems are characterised and are deeply influenced by specific national traditions. Within the broader European structure in a climate of economic and social change EU member states can be influenced by European policies. This may be one reason why Ireland, despite its conservatism was willing to participate in European educational policies, and could have had an influence on policymakers.

Horner, Dorbert et al (2007) state that

> *"Today economic, social and cultural change strengthens the need for policy makers, business leaders and scholars to learn more about the characteristics of national education systems", (2007 Pg. 1).*

They refer not only to compulsory childhood education but adult learning such as higher education and continuing or further education. Within Europe there have been many changes in the last decade with the enlargement of the EU leading to a broader focus on internationalisation and globalisation within social, cultural and educational contexts. They write that there is growing interest within Europe on education policy and policy making. This has become more topical and relevant *"due to the internationalisation of education and education studies within the overall process of globalisation"* Ibid.

They describe comparative education systems within the European context and offer an analysis of the different systems of education within the EU. They suggest that EU policy has been considerate of the many systems of education within its member states and there has been an acknowledgement of the different social, traditional and cultural backgrounds of its member states from a base of agreed principles. The stated concept is *"unity in diversity"* and the necessity to have a full understanding of the diverse member state policies and education systems before unity can be applied across the different systems. They discuss a *"systemic frame which focuses on patterns of explanatory data"* and the necessity of a comparative framework to understand the social and cultural differences of the different systems across the European spectrum.

Nevertheless within the EU, sovereign member states agree to discuss and cooperate on a range of policies, including systems of education for adult learners. In this context the broad EU policies and recommendations which emerge from engagement with member states should traverse individual national systems so that new ideas of internationalisation and globalisation can gain some traction within the EU and therefore feed back into the policies of their national members. However despite this some countries remain within traditional national policy boundaries and have not fully embraced stated EU policy on equity, inclusion and routes of access for adult learners in their choices of further or higher education.

An EU policy document produced by the Education, Audio visual and Culture Executive Agency in 2011 stated that "Adult learning opportunities are essential to ensure economic and social progress, as well as the personal fulfilment of individuals", EU(2011 Pg. 1). This agency wrote about European thinking on lifelong learning, the necessity for access and the benefits for both the individual learner, in whatever European country they were, but also the broader benefit to their society and culture and ultimately European society. Not only would opening access routes for continuing, further or higher education to adults improve European society as a whole but it would enhance employment opportunities and improvements while reflecting EU thinking and stated policies on lifelong learning for its citizens.

In 2009 the Council of the European Union agreed five targets in education and training, as part of a strategic framework for European Cooperation in Education, one of which was by 2010 to have at least 12.5% of adults across the EU member states taking part in adult education and lifelong learning. This was to be increased to 15% of adults in further education by 2020, EU (2009). The European Commission's Publication 'It is never too late to learn' , EU Commission (2006) highlighted "the essential contribution of adult education and training to competitiveness, employability and social inclusion", EU (2011). This was part of the discourse and committee work on agreements and comparisons of adult education within member states. This resulted in a European Commission Action Plan on Adult Education and Learning entitled 'It is always a good time to learn' (European Commission, 2007), This was part of a sporadic but continuous part of the EU plans of action on adult learning within its member states.

The Action Plan had specific goals and focused on the following 5 targets.

1. To analyse the effect of reforms in all sectors of education and training on adult learning;

2. To improve the quality of provision in the adult learning sector;

3. To increase the opportunities for adults to achieve a qualification at least one level higher than before (to go 'one step up');

4. To speed up the process of assessment of skills and social competences and their validation and recognition in terms of learning outcomes;

5. To improve the monitoring of the adult learning sector. EU (2007 Pg. 5).

The Irish Government's position on lifelong learning was set out in the National Plan for Equity of Access to Higher Education 2008-2013. It defined mature students as being over 23 years of age and above and set a target to increase the proportion of full-time mature students in higher education from 13 %, in 2006, to 20 % by 2013". This National Plan for Equity and Access also described the then Higher Education Authority's commitment to adult learning, further and higher education and broader routes to access higher education. They stated *"The key objective of this plan is to mainstream our approaches to improving access to higher education as in all developed countries"* HEA (2008 Pg.8) It is not clear why within the national plan, the focus was on higher education and there was no reference to a broader lifelong learning context, as advocated by the OECD in its stated principles of acknowledgement of all learning, referred to in an earlier paragraph.

The necessity of focusing on education to up skill adult learners to meet labour market needs was described in the plan. Inequity in terms of routes to access was also a significant aspect of the discussion on routes to access.

> *"all countries struggle with the challenges of inequality in education. Despite the enormous potential of education for counteracting inequality and poverty, education systems tend towards a reproduction of existing inequalities in the wider society. The inequalities that exist in education systems are most apparent in higher education"(Pg.11)*

The principles of equity and routes of access were deliberated and discussed within this publication in terms of disabilities and social economic categories, but no other areas of exclusion were discussed. This is significant as the whole CAM sector of adult learners, taking part in the many CAM training programmes have

33

been excluded from routes of access to further and higher education in Ireland. The exclusion of this sector had not been considered in this document.

1.5. Analysing Education Systems

International benchmarks for the analysis of educational systems in terms of structural frameworks with agreed analytical tools could be useful in positioning the CAM education sector within international principles of recognition of lifelong learning and the Irish National Framework of Awards. UNESCO (United Nations Educational Scientific and Cultural Organisation) designed a systems analytical tool to provide a structure for countries to assess their education systems. It is called General Education Quality Analysis/Diagnosis Framework GEQAF. UNESCO website homepage.(2014)

> *"GEQAF is structured around key elements that are proven to interactively and iteratively work together to enable the system to optimally provide quality education and effective learning experiences" (Pg. 6)*

The role of this system was to assist member countries in strengthening their capacity in assessing their education systems in terms *"of local knowledge and expertise"*, ibid.

The development of the system required the participation of member governments, and although used in childhood education at first and second levels, two of the fifteen analytical tools are arguably relevant to adult and higher education systems in Ireland. They are the tools relating to Relevance and Equity and Inclusion. Ibid These are basic principles which underpin government initiatives across the OECD and the EU and to which Ireland has committed themselves under various OECD and EU initiatives and they could have relevance in the context of CAM training provision in Ireland.

UNESCO quality framework describes lifelong learning as a necessary process to enable individuals and their societies to become sustainable, and it advocates the facilitation of continuous learning in any setting.

"An individual will not be able to meet life challenges unless he or she becomes a lifelong learner, and societies will not be sustainable unless they become learning societies. Lifelong learning has been accepted by UNESCO Member States as the master concept and guiding principle towards a viable and sustainable future. The quality of education is not only determined by formal schooling, but also by continuous provision of learning opportunities in non-formal and informal settings" Ibid,(Pg. 17)

These principles mirror those of the EU and the OECD in terms of lifelong learning and the relevance to the economic and social progress of all societies, including Ireland. The analytical tool of relevance is described by GEQAG as being country relevant in terms of work responsiveness.

Analytical Tool on Relevance: Country level relevance; Labour market and world of work responsiveness; Global level relevance; Individual level responsiveness; Internal system coherence. UNESCO website homepage.(2012)

As there is a consistent demand for education and training within the Complementary and Alternative Medicine sector within Ireland, which feeds into the labour market and is mirrored in countries internationally, it is appropriate that these principles could be adopted by Irish government bodies to acknowledge and design a framework for education and training within the CAM sector. As this demand is mirrored internationally with a public demand for therapists and treatments within the context of similar communities there is a global relevance for education and training within this sector.

Tool on Equity and Inclusion: Understanding inequity and exclusion; Policies and strategies to address inequity and exclusion", Ibid.

This second analytical tool is of particular relevance to the CAM sector in Ireland as in the Ireland of 2014 this sector, remains excluded from validation of their courses by QQI (Qualifications and Quality Ireland). This body is the custodian of the Irish National Framework of Qualifications. According to the agreed principles of inclusion and equity within the OECD and EU member states, no sector should be excluded from definition and acknowledgement of their education and practice. Citizens seeking training as part of lifelong learning should not be excluded from official policies on adult education and by definition the guidance and support which all adult learners should be able to access as part of policies of inclusion and equality.

This is not however the case, as the CAM sector is excluded from the Irish government policies relating to the acknowledgement and recognition of their training courses. All applications for validation of their courses have been suspended since 2010 and remain suspended (HETAC 2010). There is no engagement between QQI and the CAM community with regard to a lifting of this suspension and the provision of a route to acknowledgement and recognition through academic validation of education and training courses for any complementary therapy course in Ireland. Regardless of rationale a decision was taken by first HETAC and subsequently QQI to remove a route to validation of education and training for the CAM sector from the National Framework of Qualifications. The stated rationale, at the time, was that, there should be a policy framework for the recognition and regulation of the CAM by government agencies, and the DOHC (Department of Health and Children) before this suspension to academic validation could be lifted. There is further discussion on the topic in paragraph 1.10 which follows.

It could be argued that until government policy makers in Ireland and within the EU make a decision as to how to place the sector within their national policies, those responsible for recognition of education and adult learning do not have a framework to use in terms of recognition of learning. It also could be argued that the CAM sector is not a strong political lobby within Ireland and have not yet been able to make a successful case for action by government, in Ireland and in the EU.

1.5.1 AONTAS and Adult Education in Ireland

Within the broader context of adult education, the historical background of further education and adult education in Ireland can be traced back at least in part to the emergence of AONTAS in the 1960s. AONTAS an acronym for the Irish words Aos Oideachais Naisiunta Tri Aontu Soarlach, meaning 'National Adult Education Through Voluntary Unification', commenced its activities in 1969 as one of the first national initiatives in adult education. Principally involved in adult literacy, it drafted its constitution in 1970 and one of its principal goals was *"inclusiveness"* AONTAS website (2014). The commencement of AONTAS was followed by the establishment of a research committee by the then Minister of Education Brian Lenehan TD, which produced the first report on the status of adult education in Ireland. According to Kavanagh (2007) adult education was described in the Murphy Report as

> *"the provision and utilisation of facilities whereby those who are no longer participants in the full-time school system may learn whatever they need to learn at any period of their lives",* *(Pg.1).*

This report reflected a changing society in Ireland of the 1970s when adults for whatever reason began to seek *"knowledge, skills and training"* in areas they had not previously acquired within the schools system of the time. There could be many reasons for the changes in population needs within Irish society, but there is no doubt that attitudes were changing, and there was a need for the provision of learning for adult learners. The vocational education system took a leading role in offering adult learning in skills and competencies and this was a popular route to adult or further education at the time. In 2000 a White Paper was published, described as Ireland`s first

White Paper on Adult Education which adopted the principles of lifelong learning as a *"governing principle of educational policy"*, Ibid"(Pg.1).

The report was not intended to provide a structural template for adult learning but it did set out government policies and priorities at the time, one of which was

> *"to ensure that learners can move progressively and incrementally within an over-arching coordinated and learner-centred framework"*. *The Paper described adult education as "systematic learning undertaken by adults who return to learning having concluded initial education or training"*, Ibid.

This was official acknowledgement of the need for a learner centred framework which would allow adult learners to progress through a coordinated process. It was the beginning of the process of inclusion for private Learning Providers within the National Framework of Qualifications. Shortly after the publication of this White Paper, HETAC and FETAC began a process of consultation with private Learning Providers in all sectors. At this time the CAM sector was included in these consultations and in 2004 HETAC officials consulted with the National Working Group for the Regulation of Complementary Therapists, DOHC (2005). It was later, in 2010 that HETAC suspended academic validation for all CAM programmes, and stopped accepting applications for validation, HETAC (2011). This is referred to in more detail in the following paragraph.

1.6 Government and the CAM sector. Academic Validation of Training

As already stated recognition of the Complementary and Alternative Medicine community as a healthcare sector has been linked by both the Department for Health and Children and the QQI (formerly HETAC, FETAC and the NQAI) to the removal of the suspension of academic validation for CAM training. (HETAC 2010). The Department of Health's failure to define a framework or structure for this sector has been given as the reason why QQI "cannot validate CAM courses" and such courses are excluded from the National Framework of Qualifications, Ibid. This is a relatively new impasse, as prior to 2008 HETAC were fully involved with CAM learning providers in establishing quality assurance protocols as part of the application process and route to validation of courses in complementary therapies. This was their responsibility under The Qualifications (Education & Training) Act 1999. No exceptions to validation of courses from any sector were specified in the Act, up to the suspension of one CAM training programme in 2008 and the sector exclusion from the validation process in 2010.

Under the provisions of this Act, in 2003 HETAC had adopted a generic awards standard used to determine knowledge, skills and competence to be acquired by learners which would enable HETAC validate courses in Higher Education according to the National Framework of Awards.

In November 2003, HETAC adopted the generic award-type descriptors of the National Framework of Qualifications (NFQ) as Interim Standards, for the purpose of developing programmes.

Standards for Complementary Therapies have now been developed. These are an elaboration of the generic descriptors of the NFQ"HETAC (2008 Pg.1)

A small number of CAM Learning Providers had progressed through the Quality Assurance approval and validation stage of their programmes according to the 1999 Act.

.

"HETAC has agreed that as part of a pilot study relating to complementary therapy, it will initially validate programmes in three areas, namely, Acupuncture, Herbal Medicine and Traditional Chinese Medicine" , Ibid.

40

One CAM Learning Provider who had met all of the requirements and had passed all stages of the validation assessment process was notified that completion of the validation of their course was being suspended until the Department of Health agreed a process of regulation. Despite an appeal to this suspension to completion of validation, all other CAM Learning Providers were also suspended and the route to validation of their courses closed to them.

> *"As published in June 2010, the Higher Education and Training Awards Council (HETAC) formally suspended the validation of programmes in the areas of complementary therapies, pending the completion of a review, jointly commissioned by HETAC and the Department of Health and Children (DOHC), on the regulation and academic recognition of five specific therapies", (HETAC (2011).*

This review subsequently took place and a report was published in 2012. This report is reviewed within the literature review. The complementary therapy sector was given the opportunity to comment on the report. The five therapies specified in the review, Acupuncturists, Chinese Medicine Practitioners, Herbalists, Chiropractors, and Osteopaths, formed an alliance to consult on their position regarding a response to this review. A joint response to the review was made to both HETAC and the DOHC as well as individual responses from each discipline. All responses called for a lifting of the suspension of access to validation for courses in Complementary Therapies as the report had supported the sector position that it was not necessary to have one Professional Association per discipline, a reason previously given by the DOHC for their failure to agree a structure for the Complementary and Alternative Medical sector. There has been no official response from either HETAC and QQI and access to academic validation of courses in complementary therapies remains closed.

Ireland is not the only country who has not yet put in place frameworks for definition and recognition of its CAM sectors. Other

OECD and EU members such as the UK and several other European countries have a similar lack of government registration and recognition of their CAM communities. Most OECD and EU countries have informal voluntary self-regulation through Professional Associations, which do not have government oversight or support.

> *"Some governments have commissioned expert groups to investigate mechanisms for regulation of the sector and make recommendations. Ireland and the UK are among the countries who have conducted research into designing regulatory structures for CAM therapies, but who have failed to act on the recommendations of their own expert committees." Ward (2009 Pg.78).*

1.6.1 Voluntary Self -Regulation of CAM Therapies

As previously stated Complementary and Alternative Medicine is not included in any governmental structures nor is it acknowledged or recognised by the Department of Health and Children as a healthcare activity. There are no statutory regulatory structures for any CAM therapy, and no government or "official" oversight on the training, regulation or practice of complementary therapies. To fill this regulation gap, Professional Associations have emerged from the different disciplines to professionally regulate their members. The professional associations have developed Professional Codes of Ethics and Best Practice, which they report meet best international professional standards. Public information and a register of therapists are available from their websites in all disciplines. For example

> *"FICTA (Federation of Irish Complementary Therapy Associations) champions the common interests of complementary therapists and alternative medicine*

practitioners in Ireland. The federation provides a neutral and dynamic forum in which its member can meet to discuss issues of common interest or concern, and collaborate in addressing such issues to the benefit of the Complementary and Alternative Medicine (CAM) sector", FICTA website (2014).

Regulation of therapies is left to Professional Associations who have developed their own training and practice standards, and models of self-regulation for their own members. They have established and maintained professional indemnity and public liability insurance blocks for the benefit of the public and their members. They have agreed professional training and practice standards for their members and put them into practice in their membership requirements. For example

"OCI (Osteopathy Council of Ireland) aims to be the competent authority for Osteopathy in Ireland. OCI wishes to protect Osteopathy by adhering to the highest clinical and professional European and International standards until full regulation is in place. Do you want to be a member?, Osteopathy Council Website (2014).

Associations are self- funding, mostly by member subscriptions and organise their activities on a voluntary basis. Although they maintain a register of compliant members they have no statutory powers, and cannot compel therapists to join the associations or accept regulation.

An interview respondent commenting on professional regulation in a recent study said "I think we need something with teeth", Ward (2009 Pg. 68).

The only National Agencies who have consulted with some CAM Therapies, through their representative organisations and examined their policies, training and practice standards are the Health Insurance Providers in Ireland, who recognise these therapies as healthcare options for their members. BUPA on entering the Irish Health Insurance marketplace in the mid- 90s, contacted the various CAM organisations and asked them to submit information on their therapies and documentation on their training and practice standards. Once satisfied as to the professional informal regulation structures, BUPA in Ireland, began to offer rebates to its members for a small number of CAM treatments, including Acupuncture, Osteopathy, Reflexology and other therapies they considered to have professional quality oversight. VHI followed BUPA with the offer of patient treatment rebates, and this is carried on by remaining Health Insurance bodies currently in the market. On a de facto basis, the only external quality process for some CAM therapies within Ireland is commercially driven, through the Health Insurance Providers. This is also the case in both Holland and Brazil according to sector representatives interviewed for this study and documented in a later chapter.

"Professional associations in several disciplines have secured treatment rebates from all of the private healthcare providers giving patients a choice of treatment. This does not go far enough, as practitioners are not considered to be "healthcare professionals" by the Revenue Commissioners in Ireland and VAT (Value added tax) [i] *must be charged on treatments as they are considered to be providing a "service" rather than a treatment", Ibid (Pg.15).*

Conclusion

This chapter has outlined the background, context and rationale of this study. It has described chapter contents and explained the discussions within the various chapters. The chapter discussed Ireland's position and activity within the EU and OECD and how this may influence policies on acknowledgment and recognition of all forms of lifelong learning. It described the beginnings of Adult and Lifelong learning in Ireland within the broader EU context. The complementary therapy sector was defined and explained in terms of the historical context of public demand, therapy training and practice. Irish government agency policies on the regulation and academic validation of CAM training and practice has been described within the context of Ireland's membership of the EU and the OECD. The absence of academic validation of CAM training programmes and recognition of adult learning within Ireland for the CAM sector was explained. Professional voluntary self-regulatory professional structures were defined within the context of quality oversight and public safety. Finally it has noted the author's statement of interest.

Chapter 2 Literature Review

2.1 Introduction

This chapter outlines the Literature on all aspects of CAM training and practice relevant to the research questions. The literature in this review has been chosen to shed light on all aspects of CAM therapies in Ireland and in the wider EU. It explores the literature on popularity and growth of CAM, the regulation of the sector and obstacles to progress. It examines publications on healthcare in Ireland and discusses how CAM can find its place within the healthcare community and CAM training programmes within the Irish Higher Education sector. It explores the culture of quality evaluation, the marketisation and commercialisation of education. Finally it maps the National Framework of Qualifications and discusses how this could be a guide for the academic validation of CAM courses.

Hart advocates that

> *"Reviewing the literature on a topic can provide an academically enriching experience. To achieve this, the review should be regarded as a process fundamental to any worthwhile research or development work in any subject, irrespective of the discipline. The review forms the foundation of the research proper. The researcher needs to know what the contributions of others have made the knowledge pool relevant to the topic, Hart (2008, Pg. 26).*

In exploring texts and publications relevant to all aspects of this research study the following databases were searched, (PUBMED, JSTOR, AMED, ERIC, MEDLINE, EBSCO, OVID, and CINAHL). Although the literature search brought up many results, many were discarded after reading study abstracts which appeared to be of no specific relevance to the research question.

This chapter examines literature on the following subjects.

• CAM Therapies popularity and growth in Ireland and in the EU
• Regulation of CAM therapies in the EU with a focus on Ireland
• Obstacles to recognition and regulation of CAM Therapies
• Quality Assurance and reform of adult and higher education programmes in the EU with a focus on Ireland
• Consumer choice and marketisation of education
• Mapping the Irish National Framework of Qualifications

Table 2.1: Subjects Being Reviewed for Literature Review

2.2 CAM therapies popularity and growth in Ireland and in the EU

The popularity of CAM therapies in Ireland has been touched on in the opening chapter as this is fundamental to this study, and it will be discussed in this literature review in terms of the amounts of money spent on CAM treatments, in Ireland and the EU, and in terms of a shift in public social and healthcare needs. Significant amounts of money are being paid for a range of CAM treatments, which illustrates a need and demand for these therapies. An Irish CAM Professional Association report that 27 million Euros are spent each year, on one discipline alone (AFPA 2013), and patients are visiting private clinics in both urban and rural areas of Ireland to seek treatments. Irish people of all ages and backgrounds actively seek CAM therapies for a variety of disorders, (Ibid). There is also a broad use of CAM therapies as part of a regular healthcare and preventative healthcare regime. This is paralleled in countries across the world. Popularity and use of these therapies was discussed in the Irish National Working Group Report for the Regulation of Complementary Therapists.

According to this report, CAM therapies were becoming available within conventional healthcare settings.

"It is widely accepted that there has been a large increase in the number of people using complementary therapies, here in Ireland and worldwide",DOHC Report (2005,Pg. 7, Pg. 16).

The historical context of natural therapies in Ireland has been introduced in the opening chapter and historical and cultural records show there is a long history of natural healing in Ireland. Seeking cures from whatever source they are perceived to be is part of our social and cultural history. It is recorded that St Brigid, one of Ireland's patron saints who lived in the years 423 to 525 was said to have healing powers and to use natural herbs and blessings for curing a range of ailments at the time, Phillips (2004). Bonesetters and seventh sons were regularly consulted for a range of ailments. Minor common ailments were treated in rural households by naturally grown plants and herbs, such as dandelion, nettles and dock leaves.

2.2.1 Traditional Medicines

Ireland is not alone in the use of natural and self-healing, as many countries acknowledge their own traditional medicines WHO (2005) The World Health Organisation describes Traditional Medicine with reference to historical and cultural use in the countries where these practices occur.

> "..the sum total of the knowledge, skills and practices based on the theories, beliefs and experiences indigenous to different cultures, whether explicable or not, used in the maintenance of health, as well as in the prevention, diagnosis, improvement or treatment of physical and mental illnesses", WHO(2000 Pg. 134).

An international research project to record and map traditional medicine and CAM use in the developed world in terms of policy, education, research practice and use. was carried out by the WHO. This resulted in the publication of the WHO Global Atlas of Traditional, Complementary and Alternative medicine in 2005. This study was an acknowledgement of the increased use of traditional medicines and CAM therapies in the industrialised countries. One of their recommendations was that WHO member states should assist each other in developing structures and frameworks for Traditional Medicines and CAM therapies. They state that

"The use of herbal medicines and complementary and alternative medicine is increasing in industrialised countries, in connection with disease prevention and the maintenance of health. There is an emphasis on self-empowerment and a more holistic approach, in which life is understood as being a union of body, mind and soul, and health as being a combination of physical, social and spiritual wellbeing. This approach is consistent with WHOs definition of health". Ong et al (2005,Pg. 10).

Paulo Sarsina writing about the CAM or non-conventional medicine sector in Italy, in his paper *"The Social Demand for A Medicine Focused on the Person"* asserts that the need for self-empowerment and individual respect is a trend *wider than the CAM sector*, that is part of a wider social and cultural reform and it "He writes about the financial outlay for non conventional medicines in Italy and the demand from both genders, and all ages for these therapies as being part of social change. He writes

"Non Conventional Medicines have a greater social impact and the demand for such treatments of more than 10 million Italian citizens (male and female) of all ages and social classes and of thousands of Italian families reveals an interest proving that there this is a trend reversal, Ibid.

He suggests that the focus of healthcare is shifting from a "*symptom to the whole person*" Ibid. Consideration of holism within healthcare is being demonstrated as a need of the consumer or patient by the increased use of CAM therapies in many societies. Holism as a philosophy, and the consideration of the person with the illness, and how that illness impacts on the person, rather than the isolation of the illness is the basis of how most CAM therapies function. Sarsina writes

"The results of numerous surveys on health care quality carried out in the USA, in Europe and more recently in Italy show that, if a patient is asked to assess the quality of the medical treatments, his/her priorities are: humanization,

49

tailoring of the treatments, the need of attention from Public Institutions and adequate information in a comfortable environment for a free choice of the individual", Ibid.

2.3 European Research into the CAM Sector

Research into the CAM sector in Europe is limited, as there have been few studies carried out. The exception to this is the CAMbrella research project which was part funded by the EU and intended to examine the CAM sector within the Union. The project included a network of scientists across Europe who carried out eight studies under this umbrella, each participating scientist working on separate but relating subjects described as "Work Packages". Their remit included the examination of citizen demand and use of CAM, legal status of CAM in Europe, the public's perspective, the provider's perspective, and CAM research within the EU. This study was unique in that it was the first, and remains the only Pan European study with a cross European remit, into the European CAM sector. 39 countries within Europe contributed to the study with data collected from each country. Eight papers were published as part of this overall study project by the participating scientists, each documenting their own section of research. This literature review has included quotations and references from the CAMbrella project reports and some of the project findings have also been touched on within the opening chapter, as they are all relevant to public demand, need and the growth of this sector.

The project produced figures for both medical and non-medical CAM practitioners within Europe. They concluded that there are more than 150.000 medical doctors with additional CAM certification, and more than 180,000 registered and certified non-medical CAM practitioners treating a range of medical conditions within the EU. This gives the estimated figure of 330,000 medical and non-medical providers of CAM therapies in the EU. The CAM providers, both medical and non-medical deliver a comprehensive health or therapeutic service, according to figures issued by CAMbrella. (www.CAMbrella.eu).

> *"65 CAM providers per 100,000 inhabitants and 95 general medical practitioners per 100,000 inhabitants", CAMbrella website homepage.*

The project terms of reference was set out in the CAMbrella Roadmap of CAM European Research, project explanation document

> `The key areas under examination in CAMbrella had been the prevalence of CAM use, CAM terminology and definitions, citizens' needs and demands, definitions, patients' and providers' perspectives regarding CAM use, the global perspective, CAM's legal status and the drawing up of the Roadmap itself", CAMbrella (2012, Pg. 10).*

Professor Helle Johannessen Professor of Social Studies in Health and Medicine, Institute of Public Health, Faculty of Health Sciences, University of Southern Denmark, led Work Package No 3 for the CAMbrella project. She was a speaker at a conference hosted by the European Parliament and EUROCAM in 2012, and spoke about her findings as part of the CAMbrella project. EUROCAM is a European CAM alliance of organisations of patients and practitioner.

She said in relation to her findings

> *"Up to 80% of citizens in the EU Member States have used complementary and Alternative Medicines in their health care. Their hopes are to get relief from concerns that the conventional medical services do not meet and to improve general wellbeing. And yet, access to CAM, with rare exceptions, is limited to those who can afford to pay for it", CAMbrella WP2 (2012 Pg. 2).*

Patient wellbeing was a common thread which emerged from her study and was also discussed earlier in this chapter by

Sarsina.(2007). At the conference, Johannessen expanded on her findings in relation to patient needs which she had examined as her part of the CAMbrella project. She advocated that patients do not differentiate between medically trained CAM providers or non-medically trained CAM providers and said they indicated a need for wider access and therapy specific CAM providers. She said

> *"Citizens in the EU wish to have access to increased and diverse CAM provision: Studies indicate that citizens wish CAM to be available as part of their options for health care, for example in hospital and general practice care. They also wish CAM provision to be delivered not only by medical doctors and/or doctors trained in CAM specialities, nurses or other conventional health care providers, but also by CAM providers with therapy specific training. There is a wish for more, and more diverse, CAM provision", Cambrella WP3 (2012 Pg. 23).*

Growth of CAM use has been shown to be consistent in several EU countries as described by EU CAM experts at the 2012 EUROCAM Conference which took place in Brussels. One of the speakers at the conference was Dr. Harald Walach, Professor of Research Methodology and Complementary Medicine, European University Viadrina, Frankfurt/Oder, Germany, who spoke about growth and GDP of CAM within Europe. He suggested that while there is a demand for CAM therapies, there is a need for national structural regulatory frameworks, and the need for guidance and resources from the EU for its member states. He said.

> *"The growth potential of the sector, both in terms of GDP, savings on healthcare, healthier citizens, CAM workforce and innovative competitiveness is enormous. For this to happen, we need the EU to give it its due consideration and adequate resources, as well as a framework for professionals to operate in", CAMbrella (2012 Pg. 2).*

UK Prof George Lewith, of the University of Southampton who had led the CAMbrella project, Work Package 4 had carried out a systemic review of 87 previous studies pertaining to CAM use and quality assessment criteria in Europe. He reported that EU citizens chose CAM therapies as they had reported they experienced *"dissatisfaction or disappointment with a medical doctor or western medicine "*, CAMbrella (WP4 2012, Pg. 16) They also did not wish to *"take medical drugs"* and did not wish to have the side effects of drugs *"preferring natural methods"* (Ibid). Personal wellbeing and the need for an interested practitioner with whom they had a *"good therapeutic relationship"* with was described by Lewith in his paper as being important to those who chose CAM treatments.

2.3.1 CAM Research in the UK

Public behavioural change from traditional healthcare needs and public expenditure on CAM therapies was also being studied in the UK. Research studies exploring the popularity of complementary therapies among patients seeking relief for a variety of disorders. were carried out in various universities. Typically this research was quantitative, using surveys as the research tool. Two examples of these studies are the Thomas, Nicholls and Coleman (1998) study published in the journal "Complementary Therapies in Medicine" and Ernst and White (2000).

The Thomas & Coleman 1998 study was a population based survey that found that *"complementary medicine use is a substantial and growing part of healthcare behaviour"* (Pg. 156). Six named complementary therapies were included in the survey and the study showed that an estimated 22 million visits were made across the six named CAM therapies in the UK. The therapies studied were (Acupuncture, Chiropractic, Homoeopathy, Hypnotherapy, Medical Herbalism, Osteopathy). Although the NHS (National Health Service) funded 10 per cent of these visits, another 450 million pounds was paid directly by patients themselves. This was sufficient for the study to state that there was substantial use of CAM in primary healthcare.

More recently in 2009 a qualitative study was carried out in both London and Dublin where in depth interviews of patients who actively sought and paid for Complementary Medicine treatments in both cities was conducted. This study was conducted by the author to meet the requirements of the Master of Science programme at London's Middlesex University. Study data was collected from interviews by both Irish and UK CAM patients and practitioners. Patients from all walks of life seeking and paying for healthcare treatments in Ireland is not unusual, however it is significant in the UK where the National Health Service provides free healthcare. Therapies investigated in this study were Acupuncture and Chinese Medicine. Study results provide a still current snapshot of the continued need for CAM treatments in both the UK and Ireland.

> "The results of the study showed that Acupuncturists and Chinese medicine practitioners provide an effective health service, much in demand, which fills a gap and takes pressure off the systems in both the UK and Ireland", Ward (2009 Pg. 5).

The study found that the public will go to great lengths to find CAM treatments regardless of a lack of government registers of approved practitioners. As discussed by Sarsina, earlier in this chapter, this demonstrates a need for personal control and the freedom of individuals to make their own healthcare choices.

> "They want access to effective treatments from a controlled safe source. If it is not available from a safe source they will continue to seek it anyway", Ibid (Pg. 70).

Chandola, Young, McAllister and Axford writing in the Journal of the Royal Society of Medicine, conducted a survey on patients attending rheumatology and musculoskeletal clinics who used complementary therapies. 166 patients, with a diagnosis of rheumatoid arthritis took part in a structured survey questioning interest and use of therapies other than conventional therapies. 38% of those surveyed had considered the use of complementary therapies, and 28% had received a CAM therapy. 55% of those who had used complementary therapy reported gaining some benefit. The most popular therapies used were Acupuncture, Homoeopathy, Osteopathy and Herbal Medicine, with a dominance of female patients, who had expressed dissatisfaction with their medical treatments. The study demonstrated that *"Patients demand for complementary therapies cannot be ignored"* Chandola et al(1999, Pg. 13).

Similarly a survey of patients attending the out patients department of the Royal London Homoeopathic hospital was carried out in 2003 with a focus of CAM use and effect and *"to examine patients use of complementary and alternative medicine within the NHS"* Sharples, Van Haselan and Fisher (2003). 500 patients were surveyed as part of this study, which also examined the medical conditions patients suffered from as well as the duration of their condition. This hospital is a NHS facility dedicated to CAM. Of those surveyed a high number, 90% reported satisfaction with clinical care at the hospital. 81% reported that their *"clinical problem had improved very much"*, Ibid. The study concluded that conventional medicine *"is not meeting the needs of some patients and that CAM may wholly or partly be a substitute for conventional medicine"*, Ibid.

The literature demonstrates that there is popular demand for a range of CAM treatments in Ireland, the UK and within the EU. Consumer demand is consistent and manifests a steady growth of patients seeking and paying for CAM treatments, creating a demand for highly trained and safe therapists. Wellbeing, a good therapeutic relationship and the need to choose their own treatments are important to health consumers.

2.4 Regulation of CAM Therapies in the EU with reference to Ireland

The regulation of CAM therapies in Ireland has been discussed in some detail in Chapter 1, this Chapter has reviewed the literature within the broader context of regulation of CAM therapies within the EU, and discusses Irish government initiatives on consultation and the examination of a need for regulation of CAM therapies.

The EU funded CAMbrella study section on the Regulation of CAM therapies was conducted by Prof Dr Vinjar Fonnebo. She reported that of the 39 countries studied in Europe, there is no common approach to regulation of CAM, and the European Union have a "hands off" approach to CAM regulation. In her report from her section of the project, she says, with reference to CAM regulation within the EU

> "That the European Union has decided that healthcare is a national responsibility and medicinal products are regulated at union level", CAMbrella WP1 (2012 Pg. 15).

She goes on to say that

> "There is no common approach to the regulation of Cam practice in Europe. Each of the 39 countries studied do it their own way", Ibid.

While there have been EU directives on medicinal products, the latest of which has impacted on the availability of herbal and homeopathic products, EC Directive (2004), the European Union has offered no guidance or policy development on regulatory structures for the CAM sector, other than to recommend that member states develop structural frameworks themselves.

2.4.1 Irish Government Initiatives on the CAM Sector

The period between 2001 and 2006 was the most active for Irish government initiatives into CAM therapies. The then government,

56

responding to a *"a period of growing interest in issues related to Complementary and Alternative Medicine (CAM) and its regulation"*, O Sullivan (2002 Pg. 1) began consultations with the sector. In 2001 a sector wide forum on the regulation of complementary therapies in Ireland was hosted by the IPA (Institute of Public Administration) at the request of the Department for Health and Children. This forum was attended by CAM practitioners and association representatives in several disciplines. These initiatives by the Institute of Public Administration followed a public statement made in the Irish Parliament the Dáil by Minister Martin in which he committed his government to establishing a system of registration for alternative and complementary therapists. Recognising issues of public safety Minister Martin acknowledged Ireland's common law traditions which allowed practitioners to practice freely without oversight or regulation.

> *"The Minister for Health and Children, Micheál Martin TD has stated in the Dáil that he is committed to the introduction of a system of state regulation for alternative and complementary therapists who work in the area of health and personal services. Official commitment to regulation was underlined in the 2001 Health Strategy, Quality and Fairness. A Health System for You", Ibid (Pg. 6).*

Following this forum, a questionnaire was sent to all attendees and known CAM organisations as part of an IPA study. It was considered that although the forum attendees were around 100 that the viewpoints of the majority of the CAM sector had been represented at the forum and within the questionnaires. O Sullivan states

> *"The IPA study nevertheless gives the views of a significant number of CAM practitioners and of associations that represent or regulate them, Ibid.*

The focus of the O Sullivan Report was on *"regulatory and policy issues in general"* (Ibid) and was intended to document and build on the sector wide consultation which had taken place at the earlier IPA forum with CAM stakeholders.

The report acknowledged the complexity of the range of CAM therapies and the difficulty of deciding on one definition and one system of regulation,

> *"CAM therapies are extremely varied and complex and are practised by a very wide range of practitioners so it would be very difficult to find a totally satisfactory, all-encompassing definition", Ibid.*

These government initiatives on the exploration of the regularisation of the Irish CAM sector had come about as the 2001 government had committed themselves to registration of CAM therapies and had stated this in the DOHC publication *Quality and Fairness a Health System for You.* Action 106 in this publication described the criteria for deciding on the registration of CAM therapists. DOHC (2001 Pg. 122) It outlined the criteria which a therapy would need to have in order to be included in a statutory registration scheme.

Registration of CAM Therapies would rely on the following criteria

- The evidence base for each therapy
- The educational qualifications, training and experience of therapists
- The scope of practice involved
- The protection of the public and promotion of a quality service, including the efficacy of the therapies offered.

- Regulations governing alternative therapists in other countries•
the current proposals for statutory registration of health and
social care professionals in Ireland, DOHC (2001 Pg. 122).

These initiatives gained momentum in 2003 and a National Working
Group on the Regulation of Complementary and Alternative
Therapists was established reflecting the continued interest in
regulation. *This is a period of growing interest in issues related to
Complementary and Alternative Medicine"*, DOHC (2002, Pg. 5).

Sector wide consultation had again been initiated prior to the
formation of the National Working Group by contacting all known
stakeholders to select representatives to participate in this process.
The working group was made up of representatives of all of the
CAM therapies who were organised into professional groups.

> *"There are many people to be acknowledged and thanked in
> the wider complementary sector who provided information and
> attended the consultative forum.", DOHC (2005 Pg. 5).*

Areas such as categorisation and regulation of therapists in terms of
public risk and safety, scope of practice, professional oversight of
practitioners, and efficacy of treatments were the remit of the
working group. The chairperson wrote in the introduction to the
report, with reference to the role of the working group

> *"To examine the practical steps involved in the better
> regulation of complementary therapists and to continue to
> develop the consultative process for stakeholders in the
> sector" ,DOHC (2005 Pg.11).*

On completion of the working group examination of the CAM sector
The Report on the Regulation of Complementary Therapists was
published in 2005 and was made available to the CAM sector in
2006. There were several recommendations including one that the
government should regulate the CAM sector, and that the CAM
disciplines with more than one association should federate, within an

overarching CAM Council. Education and training of therapists with independent quality oversight, linked to competence and thus public safety should be academically validated by HETAC or FETAC. One of the recommendations was that HETAC and the FETAC adopt a flexible approach to the validation of CAM training programs within the report to the Department of Health, DOHC (2005 Pg. 22).

Two facilitation days were organised by the DOHC and HETAC to further discuss the sector and to examine the possibility of the sector coming together to form a single overarching CAM council. At a facilitation day attended by the researcher, the former Chair of the National Working Group (now diseased) informed those attending that there had been a change of position by government on therapy federation, as the working group had been criticised for not being inclusive of all groups, and any future process would be open to all groups. No criteria had been established for the definition of a professional association. As a result of this open door policy ad hoc associations were established with small groups of therapists, claiming a representative position at the negotiation table.

The possibility of establishing an overarching CAM council without any structural framework or guidance from government, leaving the sector to federate themselves was doomed to failure, as there was no consensus within the sector. Therapies which had previously joined, such as Acupuncture and Herbalism separated, having now been told there was no need to federate. Therapies who had contributed to the National Working Group lobbied government for assistance and oversight to no avail. A new Minister for Health was in place and the focus on the regulation of Complementary Therapies had shifted from that stated in the 2001 *Quality and Fairness a Health System for You* publication. There has been no movement from government on regulation since that time in 2006, 2007.

2.4.2 Academic Validation of CAM Courses

Education and training of CAM therapists is directly linked to the demand and supply of CAM treatments. The provision of education and training to meet this demand for competent CAM practitioners has become a valuable area of private adult education and training across all CAM disciplines.

The training of therapists has become a significant area of fee paying training within the private higher education sector. Ernst (2002).

"Student demographic has traditionally been mature students from varied backgrounds, giving many students a second chance at higher education. There is a steady and consistent public demand for complementary and alternative (CAM) therapy treatments, across the range of therapies", Ward (2009).

Coinciding with the National Working Group activities with the CAM sector, in 2004 HETAC and FETAC, responsible for higher and further education in Ireland, began a process of preparation of a process to validate CAM courses and benchmark them against the National Framework of Qualifications. This is discussed in detail in Chapter 1, and it is referred to in this Literature review, only to confirm that there was a change of governmental policy during 2008 and this resulted in the suspension of academic validation of two CAM learning courses, who had met all of the stated requirements of the Qualifications and Training Act for validation of their courses. The reasons given to the Learning Providers, was that there was an issue of recognition of the sector by the Department for Health and Children, and HETAC were now making recognition of the sector a prerequisite for the validation of CAM courses. To respond to calls from the CAM sector to lift the suspension on academic validation of CAM programmes HETAC and the DOHC initiated an international review on the regulation and academic validation of CAM programmes. This international study was carried out by a Scottish company called SMCI Associates who had successfully tendered for the project. The study commenced in 2010 and investigated regulation status and academic validation of the primary CAM therapies internationally.

The study was based on therapies which were considered to have a good evidential background, which were Acupuncture, Chinese

Medicine, Herbalism, Chiropractic and Osteopathy. Three of those fields had been identified by the DOHC working group report (2005).as Category 1 therapies in terms of risk to the public and had been recommended for statutory regulation. Two additional fields - Osteopathy and Chiropractic - were included in the study as being relevant to the study objectives.

> *"This research should take as its primary focus five fields; the three specific complementary therapies identified by the Department of Health and Children Working Group Report – Acupuncture, Herbal Medicine and Traditional Chinese Medicine and two additional fields Osteopathy and Chiropractic", SMCI (2012 Pg. 3).*

Academic validation of CAM programmes was identified as being key to safe standards training   and ultimately safe practice.

> *"All statutory regulators and most voluntary regulators within the scope of this Review require programmes to be academically validated as well as professionally accredited – assuring that the qualification is defined in relation to the relevant national qualifications framework", SMCI (2012, Pg. 2).*

The study sought to investigate all academically validated programmes of education delivered by Higher Education Institutions in Ireland and the UK. In addition the study investigated other countries whose national education frameworks had, according to the published report *"been verified as compatible with the Bologna qualifications",* (Ibid).

The study also investigated international regulatory frameworks for CAM therapies.

A further focus of the SMCI study was an investigation of any CAM programme which had been withdrawn from higher education institutes. The report outlines this objective as part of the main study.

"To identify all academically accredited/validated programmes of higher education in the same jurisdictions, where, since 2005 validation has been withdrawn or refused or where validated provision has ceased over the last five years, and an analysis of the reasons for this, whether these be driven by academic, market, political, reputational or scientific concerns".

The primary stated objective of the study was to make recommendations to HETAC and the DOHC on criteria for removing the suspension of academic validation for this sector reopening a route to academic validation of CAM programmes.

"Drawing on the information and analysis in 1 and 2 above suggest criteria for the identification of fields which have the academic and professional maturity to warrant the academic validation of programmes by HETAC", SMCI (2012 Pg. 1).

The SMCI study identified areas of *"Professional and academic maturity"*, Ibid (Pg.7). These were new terms the CAM professions had not previously been made aware of as criteria for acknowledgement of the role of a professional association. One of the study objectives and findings published in the subsequent report was to identify ways in which individual CAM disciplines could claim professional status acceptable to government.

The report described professional CAM associations in terms of needing *"Accountable organisational structures and process and legitimate expertise "* in order to be identified eligible to claim *"professional"* status. Ibid   It listed a number of attributes a professional organisation should have in order to become *"professionally mature"*. These included such criteria as a democratic structure, published codes of ethics and practice, disciplinary code for its members and methods of enforcing it. Many of these criteria had already been met by a range of professional CAM associations, indeed they were visible on their websites, and in some cases had already been submitted to the DOHC during sector consultation which preceded the formation of the National Working

Group on the Regulation of Complementary Therapists during 2004 and 2005.

One of the recommended attributes in the SMCI report was the requirement to have an independent assessment of qualifications

"independently assessed entry qualifications (to assure that new professionals are fit to practise, SMCI (2012 Pg. 8).

The recommendations fell short of fulfilling the study`s stated objectives in making a direct recommendation to HETAC on what would be necessary to permit the academic validation of CAM courses.

Those objectives were outlined in the study rationale and were to

"suggest criteria for the identification of fields which have the academic and   professional maturity to warrant the academic validation of programmes by HETAC", SMCI (2012 Pg.1).

Instead the study laid out a set of generic guidelines in which professional bodies might achieve *"professional maturity"* without a conclusive suggestion or recommendation on the academic validation of CAM courses, which was the stated purpose of the study. It was also unclear from the SMCI report which government agency would evaluate professional maturity of the various associations, as no recommendation was made in the report regarding this and it was not addressed other than to list professional maturity as criteria for inclusion in any government programme. Subsequently no action has been taken by HETAC and the newly formed Quality and Qualifications Ireland authority (QQI) responsible for academic validation of all learning in Ireland. CAM courses remain without a route to academic validation in Ireland, (QQI website 2014). The CAM sector remains unregulated in Ireland with no government guidance or facilitation and stakeholders reportedly continue to lobby government agencies for a lifting of suspension of academic validation of training programmes.

2.4.3 Professional Accreditation in Ireland

The de facto status of voluntary professional organisations who had established themselves as self- regulatory bodies was acknowledged and supported by the working group in the registration and oversight of therapists. They argued that all therapists should be registered within a professional association "

> *"This will ensure that the public will be able to access up-to-date sources of information and make an informed judgment as to what they can expect from a competent and registered practitioner",* DOHC (2005 Pg.32).

In many disciplines such as Acupuncture, Chinese Medicine, Medical Herbalism, Homoeopathy, Chiropractic and Osteopathy, professional bodies are long established, filling a regulatory gap on a voluntary basis. In Ireland professional associations such as AFPA, (Acupuncture Foundation Professional Association), FICTA,(Federation of Irish Complementary Therapy Associations), OCI (Osteopathic Council of Ireland) and ISH (Irish Society of Homoeopaths, to name just a few of the associations, have long regulated their members and have been left to do so without any input by successive governments both in Ireland and the UK.

Government has fallen short of approving or supporting the work of the professional bodies in all disciplines and there is no compulsion for a therapist practicing any therapy to join a professional association. There are no sanctions for practitioners or therapists who choose not to belong to a professional association, and as there are no official registers the public in many cases are unaware of this lack of oversight. This translates into a significant public safety issue. The National Working Group asserted that professional associations were necessary for the registration and professional oversight of therapists.

> *"It is frequently the case that the term "complementary therapist" is inaccurately applied, usually by the media, to an untrained and/or unregistered self-styled practitioner who has come to public notice through malpractice. A sham practitioner*

or rogue trader might be a more accurate description", NWG Report (2005 Pg. 5).

2.5 Opposition to the Recognition and Regulation of CAM Therapies

There is considerable opposition by the biomedical and broad healthcare sector to any government recognition of CAM therapies and subsequently the academic validation of CAM courses. Obstacles intended to restrict, obstruct or reduce the levels of recognition for CAM therapies are common not only in Ireland but in many countries in the EU and elsewhere. The lack of "acceptable" research on CAM therapies is regularly used as a reason to deny any official recognition of CAM therapies. This argument has become less powerful with the emergence of several clinical trials demonstrating the efficacy of various CAM treatments such as Acupuncture, Herbalism and Osteopathy.

The Naturopathy Digest in an article by Alex Vasquez discussed the American Medical Association. Entitled

> *"AMA Declares War on Naturopathic Medicine, Patient Safety and Freedom of Choice in Health Care*
>
> *Behind the usual façade and overused disguise of "patient safety," "science" and "high standards," the American Medical Association (AMA) and several other allopathic (MD) medical groups are again seeking to limit the scope of practice and state licensure for other duly trained healthcare professionals",(Vasquez 2006 Pg. 2).*

According to Vasquez, the AMA are clear about their goal to obstruct and block licensures for naturopaths and chiropractors. In 2006, they placed the following statement on their website.

> *"RESOLVED, That our American Medical Association work through its Board of   Trustees to   outline a policy opposing the licensure of naturopaths to practice medicine and report this policy to the House of Delegates no later than the 2006*

Interim Meeting. (Directive to Take Action) Fiscal Note: Implement accordingly at estimated staff cost of $10,836",(Ibid).

A headline in a in the Times of London entitled *"Happy Twaddle Free Birthday to the NHS "*by Journalist Alice Miles from the Times of London and published in June 2008, cited in Ward (2009), refers to the intended formation of a UK regulation structure for Complementary Therapies

> *" the publication of the Report to Ministers from the Department of Health Steering Group on the Statutory Regulation of Practitioners of Acupuncture, Herbal Medicine, Traditional Chinese Medicine and Other Traditional Medicine Systems Practiced in the UK otherwise known as twaddle".* London Times (2008)

The article went on to describe the statutory regulation of (CAM) practitioners as *"The greatest risk to the health of the NHS"* and says that *"doctors see no scientific merit whatsoever"* in treatments and then states that Professor Edward Ernst describes the majority of CAM therapies as *"clinically ineffective"* and *"dangerous"*.

It could be argued that a blanket statement such as those stated above does not fairly represent the whole CAM sector. The 2008 UK Report to the Ministers from the Steering Group, referred only to CAM therapies which have a good evidential background and can be regarded as such to have scientific merit. This is the same criteria used by the Irish governmental reports. It is unfortunate that all CAM therapies for the purposes of this article and media response to the publication of the Report have been grouped together, and the sector judged as dangerous when only therapies with good scientific studies had been included for discussion on regulation. Another similar article authored by David Colquhoun and also published in the London Times of August 2008 was entitled *"Regulating quack medicine makes me feel sick"*. He states that these therapies should not be regulated because there is no evidence of effect.

> *"It is fashionable to think things are true for no better reason than you wish it were so. Anything goes, from fairies, crystals*

67

and Ayurvedic medicine (as advocated by Cherie Blair) to fooling yourself about WMD (as advocated by her husband ",London Times (2008).

The article continues to complain about the UK Government initiatives to form regulatory structures, complaining about the lack of evidence of effect. This too is a grouping of evidenced based CAM therapies and the weakest of trends described as CAM therapies in order to make a point. All published efforts to regulate CAM education, training and practice meet with hysterical responses from some sections of the media. . The following is a further comment in the London Times

> *"The latest sign of this trend is a report to the Department of Health from Professor Michael Pittilo, Vice-Chancellor of the Robert Gordon University, Aberdeen. His May report - on acupuncture, herbal medicine, traditional Chinese medicine and the like - recommends that these therapies should have statutory regulation run by the Health Professions Council, and that entry for practitioners should "normally be through a bachelor degree with honours".(Ibid).*

There are currently websites such as QuackWatch.com and Scepdic.com who devote considerable time, effort and finance into attacking CAM therapies. This is an extract from one example of such published attacks from the website Scepdics.com.

This has a permanent place on their website under their Dictionary entitles "*From Abracadabra to Zombies*". CAM Professional bodies report a heightening of both published and internet attacks as various governments consider regulatory strategies.

> *"The term 'complementary' seems to have been introduced by the purveyors of quackery in an attempt to produce the bias that untested or discredited treatments should be used along with scientifically tested medical treatments. There really is no such thing as "alternative" medicine; if it's medicine, it's medicine. 'Alternative medicine' is a deceptive term that tries to create the illusion that a discredited or untested treatment is truly an alternative to an established treatment in scientific medicine.*

By adding 'complementary medicine' to the repertoire of misleading terms, the purveyors of quackery have improved on the illusion that their remedies somehow enhance or improve the effects of science-based medical treatments, Scepdics.com (2014).

Most CAM professionals and their professional organisations would also advocate the necessity of evidence of effect and promote therapy practice from an evidence base, so the criticism of no evidence does not stand up in the light of current scientific studies, including Randomised Controlled Trials for several of the stronger CAM therapies. With reference to the comment of the terminology used to describe CAM therapies, the description of Complementary and Alternative Medicine is one that is in common usage for many years in many countries, and has been defined by the World Health Organisation to describe such healthcare and therapeutic practices, WHO(2005 Pg. 1). The CAM sector would argue that their healthcare and therapeutic practices are not an alternative to conventional medicine, but can complement conventional healthcare choices.

2.6. Consumer Choice

The literature on the popularity of CAM treatments demonstrates that consumers choose and pay for CAM therapies in Ireland and elsewhere. Their right to choose, despite opposition to their choices is entrenched in consumer protection rights. The right to choose any goods or service was first advocated by US President John F Kennedy when he addressed the US Congress and outlined four consumer rights.

"The right to safety, the right to be informed, the right to choose and the right to be heard", Kennedy J F (1963).

In 1981 the United Nations Economic and Social Council drafted a set of guidelines which were intended to outline and to protect consumer rights. Following extensive consultations among UN members, in April 1985 these guidelines were adopted by a consensus resolution of the United Nations General Assembly

69

Patients seeking CAM treatments, as stated, were interviewed in a qualitative study to explore the reasons why they seek out CAM treatments and pay for them when other treatments may be free. One of the findings of that study was that

> "CAM patients are informed consumers, they evaluate treatments as they go along. They attend if they get benefit and they stop when they don't", Ward (2009 Pg. 71).

The National Working Group on the Regulation of CAM Therapists found that

> "It is for the consumer to make the choice of which therapy they intend to use. Whether they wish to consult a qualified therapist such as a homeopath or an acupuncturist, a healer, the seventh son of a seventh son, a person reputed to have a cure for a particular ailment or a person with a special skill with bones; the choice is theirs", DOHC (2005 Pg. 7).

The report went on to state that "the public needed a clear source of information regarding standards to be expected." The report also stated that a register of safe competent practitioners was needed in order to protect public safety.

> "It would also be expected that the public would exercise as much care and responsibility in taking sensible, informed decisions with regard to their own health care", DOHC(2005 Pg. 8).

The literature on consumer rights demonstrates that the public have protection in law to make their own decisions as to what products and services they choose. Texts and publications confirm that members of the public cannot be presumed to be naive participants in their own lives. They have the right to inform themselves, and there is evidence they do inform themselves before making their own choices. The consumer's right to choose a healthcare treatment has become the basis of the Portuguese CAM sector government lobby for a statutory framework. This appears to have met with some success as Portugal has designed legislation for the categorisation and regulation of their CAM sector, which if passed, will become the first European country to frame such legislation.

2.7 Quality Assurance of Adult and Higher Education Ireland and Europe

The history of quality assurance frameworks and policies can be traced back to customer service goals from a world emerging from the constraints of war in the 1950s to develop the first quality models. Total quality management systems or TQM as they are known as, were developed and implemented widely across industry in the fifties and sixties. Experts such as Ishikiwa, Tagushi and Shingo initiated the early total quality models. Tsutsui WM (1996).They were followed by Tom Peters(1982) and Tom Collins (1994),(2001). The quality focus was based on customer service and satisfaction and continuous improvement in the delivery of product or service. This quality model is well accepted in retail and commercial settings however the concept, within the adult learning sector that the student, as the consumer, should be put at the centre of education planning and delivery as part of an educational quality model is a relatively new one.

The culture of evaluation and quality had been evolving in Ireland and became part of the public service and educational cultures at all levels, especially when linked to external funding, when process and results needed to be justified. In an article entitled *Contexts and Constraints An Analysis of the Evolution of Evaluation in Ireland with Particular Reference to the School Sector"* McNamara, O Hara, O Sullivan and Boyle discussed the history of the evaluation culture in Ireland. The authors traced this culture of evaluation over the past three decades to the direct influence of external bodies such as the EU and also the OECD. Initially directed to governance and the public service and based on a transparent measurement of the best use of government funds, they state that

> *"In recent years a broad quality assurance agenda within the public service and to an extent beyond has emerged",* McNamara et al (2008).

McNamara et al describe an Ireland of the seventies and eighties when there was very little external oversight on government or institutional projects and policies. They discuss the economic pressures in Ireland of the eighties when government focus was not on evaluation or quality measurement of service, but on public expenditure. It was a time of high taxation and *"good governance took a back seat against the drive to control public expenditure",* Ibid. The examination on the use of funds was not a priority at the time

The exception to this was on projects linked to EU funding where there was a formal requirement to show value for money and transparent expenditure of EU funds where a demand for evaluation was "consistent and systemic". Ibid.

> *"Ireland has been a major beneficiary of funding support from the EU. Tied to this expenditure was a requirement to evaluate EU-funded programmes", (Ibid).*

The culture of quality evaluation, first introduced to Ireland, has been directly linked to funding, became an embedded part of Irish governmental culture in the 2000s. They argue that the transference of quality culture into the educational system in a modern system of quality evaluation became an extension of government oversight in allocation of funds across all government departments.

2.7.1 Quality in Higher Education - EU Quality Framework

Quality assurance for higher education in Ireland became a focus of the Department of Education in the early 2000s. This replicated

72

events in the broader context of European higher education. The Council of Europe and the European Parliament adopted a common European higher educational quality framework in April 2008. Known as the European Quality Framework (EQF) it is based on standardisation of higher education learning outcomes across Europe, with the objectives of ease of transfer of skills and academic training within the EU to benefit travel and work within EU member countries. The Irish quality standards and quality framework is referenced to the EQF as Ireland was one of its signatories.

"In common usage, the term 'quality assurance' (QA) means 'the maintenance of a desired level of quality in a service or product, especially by means of attention to every stage of the process of delivery or production'. In essence this is the meaning it has in higher education particularly in respect of provider-owned quality assurance)", HETAC (2011).

This quality framework for the first time, acknowledged "provider owned" or private higher educational learning institutions outside of the standard university or VEC model. The development of the EQF was a model which would help to standardise learning and training and permit EU national governments to accredit such institutions and to help them to align against the National framework of Qualifications

"Provider-owned quality assurance extends to areas including teaching, assessment, curriculum, learning environment, human resources (including academic staff) health and safety, accessibility, learner support services, finance, planning, partnerships, governance, management", Ibid.

Individual learning providers prior to application for validation of training programmes were obliged to conduct a systemic audit of every aspect of their training programmes in order to draft a quality manual. The quality manuals became the working manual of management, teachers and assessors. Annual self-evaluation audits and reports became part of quality procedures.

2.7. 2 Government Reform in Higher Education

The Bologna Agreement and Declaration signed by 29 countries in Bologna Italy in July 1999, marked a turning point in higher education within Europe. With the intent of creating a general higher education framework across European signatories to allow recognition and *"convergence"* of European higher education standards. The Bologna Declaration did not seek to impose reform in higher education on member governments but to permit a method of standardisation of recognition of qualifications across Europe.

One of the principal aspects of the Bologna Agreement was the adoption of ECTS (European Credit Transfer System) to measure learning. This removed the focus from formal teaching and re focused on all methods of learning towards achieving stated learning outcomes. Ireland was one of the first 29 countries to sign the Bologna Declaration.

> *"Establishment of a system of credits - such as in the ECTS system - as a proper means of promoting the most widespread student mobility. Credits could also be acquired in non higher education contexts, including lifelong learning, provided they are recognised by the receiving universities concerned"*, Bologna (1999).

Prior to the commitment to the Bologna Declaration quality in higher education in Ireland was a stated expectation but no templates and very little provider guidance was available from HETAC or FETAC outside of the university system. The introduction of quality frameworks into higher and further education has therefore been relatively recent, and driven by the EU commission and EU European Quality Framework. HETAC and FETAC now measure quality of programme delivery, progress and improvement on their Quality frameworks. In 2011 HETAC published updated guidelines on quality assurance procedures which replaced their earlier more generic publication of 2002. (HETAC) 2011. This reflected the European Quality Framework standards and the focus was on achieving learning outcomes.

Government reform is ongoing as a Quality Assurance Bill was published in July 2011. This provided for a complete restructuring of higher education in Ireland, with the merging of the further and higher education agencies into the Qualifications and Quality Ireland (QQI).

> *"The newly formed QQI will facilitate the achievement of a coherent and consistently applied system of qualifications and quality assurance in education and training nationally. It will maintain, promote and develop the National Framework of Qualifications (NFQ), working with Institutions and providers to ensure that greater opportunities will be available to learners nationally for participation in high quality education and training",* FETAC,(2011).

The National Framework of Qualifications is the benchmark for levels of qualifications in further and higher education. Until the suspension of academic validation for the CAM sector, the NFQ was the framework which guided the academic validation of courses delivered by private providers, including those from the CAM sector. It is the level framework for all Non Irish or Non Irish validated qualifications including those from the CAM sector.

2.8 Marketisation in Education

Marketisation of higher education programmes has become embedded within governmental policy across the developed countries as higher education institutions are expected to accept financial and viability responsibility for their programmes.

Those who advocate neo liberal ideals in all contexts argue that the market will find its level on the basis of supply and demand, and actions and decisions should be taken on the basis of free market and cost. First advocated by Margaret Thatcher and Ronald Reagan who stated that the free market would give more individual choice and the removal of government oversight on many aspects of life which would empower individuals and remove a *"dependency on a nanny state"*. Thatcher and Reagan advocated privatisation of many traditional government functions to allow the free market full rein, therefore removing traditional *"burdens"* from governments.

> *"Neo liberalism is a philosophy in which the existence and operation of a market are valued in themselves, separately from any previous relationship..... The idea that everyone should be an entrepreneur is distinctly neoliberal. For neoliberals it is not sufficient that there is a market: there must be nothing which is not market"*, Fitzsimons (2002).

Within the context of education neo liberalist ideals and the commercialisation of education provision removes the sole burden of responsibility for the financing and provision of higher education from governments and puts it in the remit of the higher education institutes. The concept that the student must be regarded as the consumer and that a business model must be part of an overall management structure to manage higher education programmes has been pushed through all levels of education provision from the minister to the teacher. Programmes are expected to be in profit and no longer a drain on the university and therefore government. Higher Education institutions are expected to compete with each other and attract students to maintain their viability. The direct responsibility is therefore no longer solely left with government and education budgets but shifted within performance expectations to the institutions. According to Cardoso et al higher education institutions are

"Compelled by financial constraints and by the market logic (emphasis on efficiency, effectiveness, quality and competition), they are placed in a new inter-institutional competition where attracting students is one of the most structuring components", Cardoso, Carvalho and Santiago (2011).

Universities must find ways to market their programmes so that they remain viable. There is much criticism across the developed world at the introduction of statutory provisions in several countries which focus on the *"commercialisation of public universities"* and therefore the reduction of governmental financial responsibility".

Critics of commercialisation of higher education argue that in the rush to commercialise and market higher education programmes, academic values have been lost. They argue that access to programmes will be reduced and higher education will return to access for the privileged in society. They seek to return to traditional academic values and equality and remove the focus on finance and managerial priorities within the higher education institutions

"The regulations and their main criticisms have failed to address the underlying causes to educational inequity and the lack of emphasis on the impacts of privatisation and marketisation on academic values and purposes of higher education", Susanti, D. (2011).

Marketisation of education is not a new concept within the CAM education and training community. CAM education and training stands or falls on the commercialisation of the training programmes, as all CAM education and training in Ireland falls within the private education sector. The challenge to CAM Learning Providers to try to maintain the integrity of their course curriculum, while remaining competitive within the higher education market is considerable. Neo liberalist ideals and Marketisation of education have always been a feature of privately delivered CAM education and training at all levels. The student, as consumer chooses and evaluates the CAM training course and Learning Providers must provide for this in course planning and delivery.

2.8.1 Self Evaluation

Quality assurance procedures require ongoing self-evaluation and self- assessment and annual review. The evaluation and assessment process is an important "living" part of quality assurance protocols and is typically detailed and documented within a Quality Assurance (QA) manual. Key evaluation and assessment principles for review are detailed, and the institution functions and develops within the framework of the QA protocol. It is in effect the bible of programme managers and teachers.

McNamara and O Hara in their book *Trusting Schools and Teachers* present the argument that external inspection of schools and teaching processes is not an effective evaluation method.

"There are serious drawbacks to monitoring systems which are primarily concerned with making judgements from an external prospective", McNamara and O Hara (2008).

The authors go on to state that

"external monitoring of an intrusive kind can seriously damage the autonomy and morale of professionals and organisations",(Ibid).

They make the argument that institutions will perform better if everyone engaged in providing teaching is empowered within a system of accountability. Evidence and data from student outcomes would be used by teachers and management to self-evaluate their own work and student outcomes. This system of self-evaluation does not remove external monitoring of teaching and learning, but shifts the focus from external judgement to engaging and empowering teachers and staff into taking responsibility for their own tasks, and submitting the data, based on evidence to the external evaluators.

This resonates within the CAM community of Learning Providers, as quality, accountability and self-evaluation is now an embedded part of further and higher education. CAM Learning Providers, just as any other providers of adult education must embrace accountability and self-evaluation as a continuous quality process in the delivery of education and training. The emergence and maintenance of quality processes within adult education is part of the validation and accreditation process and while the CAM community continue to lobby government for inclusion, recognition and academic validation of their qualifications, quality processes must be in place in their education and training programmes.

> *"Quality development in higher education is often limited to bureaucratic documentation, and disregards the development of quality as an organisation's holistic culture. However, there is a need to focus on promoting a quality culture which is enabling individual actors to continuously improve educational practice", Ehlers (2009).*

2.8.2 National Framework of Qualifications (NFQ)

The newly established agency QQI (Quality and Qualifications Ireland) authority governs all routes to academic validation at all academic levels in Ireland, and has the responsibility for developing policy for their legislative duties in implementing the National Framework of Qualifications.

QQI are comprised of the of the former higher education and further education agencies. HETAC, FETAC and the NQAI, and some of their functions are to

"Promote, maintain, further develop and implement the (National) Framework of Qualifications", Education and Training Act (2012).

They validate and award academic qualifications, monitor and review learning providers. The authority also can delegate authority to make awards and has the responsibility of external quality monitoring of Irish Universities. The mapping of the NFQ is relevant to this research study as validation of training is benchmarked against the NFQ levels, as is levelling of qualifications validated externally outside of Ireland. The NFQ is a system of 10 levels of learning based on nationally agreed criteria at each level. Each level represents the learning outcomes expected of learners on completion of courses at each of the ten levels. It maps learning from the most basic to the most advanced. Each level represents an award, in recognition of the learning outcomes achieved. Major awards in the National framework represent specific names awards and Minor awards are a recognition of achieving some learning outcomes, which may not meet the criteria of a major award but are a recognition of achievement. Special purpose and supplemental awards are also listed on the NFQ and are recognition of learning, either for a specific purpose or to supplement an existing award.

The NFQ represents all learning which takes place *"in schools, colleges, at work or in the home and the community"*, QQI website (2013).

Levels 1 to 5 of the NFQ represent early learning from initial literacy and numeracy at levels 1 and 2 to completion of the Leaving Certificate at Level 5. Level 6 is mapped as an Advanced Certificate which previously was the FETAC remit and is a vocational qualification. Learners can progress to higher levels within the NFQ with additional learning. A Higher Certificate is also mapped at Level 6 on the NFQ. This was previously awarded by HETAC and learners can progress to the next level of the framework with additional learning. The framework is outlined in the following table.

Adult education is evaluated and levelled against the NFQ levels, and this is a consideration for CAM learning Providers, while planning and delivering their training programmes. Although the route to academic validation for the CAM sector is currently, closed in Ireland, the NFQ levels are a useful reference benchmark for CAM Learning Providers. The sector continues to lobby government for inclusion in the validation process and it makes sense that course planners use the NFQ levels in the self evaluation of their training programmes. Some CAM Learning Providers have been obliged to seek non Irish validation of the training programmes, and NFQ levels are relevant to the recognition in Ireland and within Europe of their non Irish qualifications.

The NFQ Levels and descriptions are outlined in the following table.

Levels 1 to 6	Common Awards System (CAS) which is intended to be implemented in the Spring of 2014.
Level 7	Ordinary Bachelor's Degree following three years study at a *"recognised higher educational institution".*(QQI website 2013). Learners can progress to a higher award on the NFQ with additional learning
Level 8	Honours Degree Programme, following completion of three years study in a *"recognised higher education institution".* Ibid. Learners can progress to Master's Degree . This award is authorised by QQI HETAC
Level 8	Higher Diploma to transfer from Level 8 to Level 9
Level 9	Masters Degree, usually accessible by learners with a Level 8 Bachelors Honours Degree, but in some cases can be accessed by learners with an Ordinary Degree This is authorised by QQI HETAC and progression is available to Level 10 of the NFQ.
Level 10	Advanced learning to a Doctoral Degree. Learners would typically have achieved an honours Bachelors degree and Masters degree in order to take part in the doctoral degree programme. The awarding body for a Doctoral Degree is QQI for HETAC awards, the universities and the Institutes of Technology.

Table 2.2: National Framework of Qualifications (NFQ)

A Higher Doctorate is also mapped at Level 10 of the NFQ. This is not a validated award or an award achieved by completing a programme of learning. It is awarded for achievement in excellence and is often awarded to a candidate who already holds a Doctorate at Level 10.

The NFQ, as stated, is the benchmark which CAM Learning Providers level and match their programmes, and would be the guiding process for academic validation of CAM education and training at all levels, as it is with other private sectors. The CAM sector, as stated, continues to lobby government and the Department of Education for a restoration of their right to apply for validation of their courses according to the National Framework of Qualifications, so CAM students could continue their education to the highest academic level in Ireland as they do in other European countries.

Conclusion

In conclusion to this literature review available texts and publications relevant to the public demand for CAM therapies demonstrating a trend for social change in Europe are outlined. Research within the UK and Europe on CAM therapies has been reviewed and discussed. Reforms in adult education and the emergence of quality processes and how they impact on the education sector are discussed. Publications on the delivery of adult and higher education and the concept that the student as consumer is key to the teaching and learning partnership is reviewed and discussed. Literature on the current Irish and European education climate within a culture of reform and quality assessment, which demands value for money, is reviewed. The relevance of educational reform within adult education and how this might impact on the CAM sector, and the study questions is discussed. There is no doubt that quality oversight and accountability can only improve the delivery of education and Ireland can take its place in the EU and the wider world in terms of quality and delivery. The review does however illustrate that the system of recognition and validation of training and a recognition of qualifications is not inclusive for paths to learning and there is still much work to be done in the area of inclusion for the CAM sector.

Chapter 3: Study Methodology

3.1 Introduction

In this chapter the study methodology considered to be the best fit to address and explore all aspects of the research questions is outlined and described. The rationale for employing a mixed methodology incorporating a model of needs analysis from within an explorative flexible paradigm is discussed and explained. Research sequencing of both the quantitative and qualitative phases of the study are presented and defined. There was no hierarchy used in the sequencing of study methods, the sequencing used made sense to the data collection chain. Key literature on all aspects of using a mixed methodology are examined and discussed. Analysis methodology philosophy and framework are described for both the quantitative and qualitative sequences of the study. The researcher also discusses the challenges in examining what is a niche specialist population of Complementary and Alternative Medicine (CAM) stakeholders within a specialist sector.

3.2 Methodological Paradigm

The methodology chosen for this study is a post positivist exploratory mixed method style of research using both quantitative and qualitative research tools. The focus of the study is a needs analysis for a niche community so an exploratory, flexible paradigm was considered to be appropriate. The study fits into the exploratory paradigm as there is very little research from within this sector and little information on sector learning providers is currently available. A mixed methods strategy was chosen to best fit the study both in terms of data collection and data analysis. Robson writes about mixed methodologies and states

" there can be considerable advantages to using mixed methods designs, that is designs which make use of two or more methods and which may yield both quantitative and qualitative data", Robson (2007, Pg. 5).

According to Greene mixed methods empirical research in the field of education is quite common, although takes a wide variety of forms from mixing different types of data collection techniques to mixing different kinds of enquiry Green (2007, Pg. 20). Denscombe writes that using different methodologies within a single study is not a new strategy as social researchers have been using mixed methodologies successfully for years. He writes that only when the term *"mixed methods approach was championed by writers such as Creswell (2009), Creswell and Plano Clark (2007), Green (2007)* "and other advocates of these strategies, that the method gained scientific respect and credibility. Denscombe (2010, Pg. 137).

The study was by necessity exploratory as previously stated, as analysis of the sector in terms of stakeholder status, function, attitudes, goals and objectives was central to the exploration of this community. This is the first study of its type in Ireland to explore this community, its past and present activities and its future objectives. Little is known about stakeholders and the detail of the provision of learning and training in this sector. Learning providers are independent and there was no information on quality oversight of any of the training programmes being delivered. There is also limited data on the methods of oversight of the practice of complementary therapies, both in Ireland and other countries with similar population needs. The study design needed to provide substantive information as to who the Complementary and Alternative Medical stakeholders were, how they operated, what their concerns, values, plans and objectives for the future were. The study also sought to explore how education and training fitted into adult or higher education in Ireland, and the status of complementary therapies within the broader healthcare sector. CAM training and practice in the UK and other countries with similar educational and healthcare structures were also included in the sample to inform the study and provide comparative data. The complementary and alternative medical sector in Ireland is a niche area which the researcher has worked in and has background knowledge of. A niche research sample is described as an area or field where the researcher is familiar or works with and has access to research in that particular niche community. *"Your niche is an exclusive corner of your field where you could conduct research"*, NIH Online (2014).

This study as it explored the detail of the function and status of complementary therapies evolved into a broader analysis of needs for this community and its many stakeholders. Gathering data on historical events or present status lent itself to the further exploration of future plans and needs. Using both quantitative and qualitative methods the research sought to identify the needs and objectives of this community in the provision of education and training to adult learners and the practice of their therapies into the future. As the professional therapist is the product of these training courses, their views and opinions were also central to an analysis of the sector. The educators, regulators and the practitioners are the major stakeholders from within this community and were central to this study.

Each section of this sector is heavily involved in the current work and future plans and is key to its survival and potential development. Their experiences and opinions from working within the sector, exploration of their goals and objectives for their future work were an important part of the study evaluation and needs analysis for this sector. The CAM community functions in what is an insecure, unsupported and unregulated environment and concerns for growth and development and their continued work are typically expressed from within this community. Data gathered as part of this study explored the attitudes, views and judgements on the current status, challenges and intentions of each of the stakeholders.

3.3 Study Methodological Framework

The conceptual framework of the research study according to Miles and Huberman (1994) is fundamental to the research study, as researcher assumptions, *"expectations and beliefs that supports and informs the study is a key part of the design".* It helps the researcher to map the study design towards answering the research questions and meeting research goals. The literature can help to inform the conceptual or theoretical framework but the study is by necessity subjective and the problem being studied will in itself guide the methodology. Miles and Huberman write that

> *"An important part of the Conceptual Framework is the identification of the philosophical or methodological paradigm the researcher chooses to inform the study",(1994 Pg. 42).*

The study, as discussed, is rooted within a post positivist qualitative paradigm. There are historical differences between the methodological paradigms in both the positivist and post positivist philosophies *"each embodying very different ideas about reality (ontology) and how we gain knowledge (epistemology)".* The positivist or as sometimes described as the scientific method of research has according to Walliman (2005,Pg. 12) been applied to research in areas which are not considered to be *"scientific* "such as sociology, psychology and education " *although some scientists question the appropriateness of doing this"*

He writes that positivism as a research method was influenced by

> *"nineteenth century empiricist thinkers such as Bacon and Hume holds that every rationally justifiable assertion can be scientifically verified or is capable of logical or mathematical proof, (Pg..16).*

> *In its simplest form positivist research is governed by quantitative mathematical principles and will deliver the "what" within a research question, while the post positivist research methodologies within qualitative research will deliver the " how and why" of the research question. Elliot et al describes qualitative research as being based in knowledge development.*

87

They write that

"the aims of the qualitative researcher is to attempt to understand and represent the experiences and will attempt to engage and describe the lived experiences of people as they encounter, engage and live through situations", Elliot et al,(1999).

A mixed methodology study using both positivist quantitative and a post positivist qualitative methodologies is intended to deliver a wider understanding of the topic being studied. Each methodology has its own intrinsic value and using both methods within a single study can add to the depth and development of subject knowledge and better answer the research questions.

As this study although explorative also fits into an interpretivist paradigm. Walliman (2008) presents *"The interpretivist alternative"* a post positivist qualitative research paradigm he describes as based on idealism and our own or others experiences, beliefs and perceptions. *"We are not neutral disembodied observers"* Ibid (Pg.. 17). Denzin and Lincoln (2003) write that the foundation or traditional period of research was associated with *"the positivist foundational paradigm"* whereas the *"modernist or golden age or blurred genres moments are connected to the post positivist arguments,* Ibid (Pg..4).

According to Greene (2007), the overall purpose of using mixed methods in a single study to gather and analyse data is *"to develop a better understanding of the phenomena being studied"* (Pg.98). She advocates that using a mix of methods as part of an empirical study will generate more comprehensive data and provide the researcher with a broader context of the data being studied. This can add research rigour and can mean *"getting it right, enhancing the validity and credibility of our findings",* (ibid).

A flexible paradigm was considered the most appropriate method of enquiry incorporating both quantitative and qualitative research elements, to allow some flexibility as the qualitative collection continues. This is especially useful within semi structured interviews, as emerging themes in early interviews can be added to a guide question list for later interviews. Robson writes that a study can develop as it is conducted, allowing the data to evolve and *"unfold as the research proceeds"*. It also, as stated, allows initial data to be revisited following analysis of early data to inform further data. The flexible design label allows a wider research context so that the research may include an ontological reality within a mixed study delivering both quantitative and qualitative data. Denscombe advocates that the *"mixed methods approach has three characteristic features which set it apart from other strategies for social research"*, Denscombe (2010 Pg. 138). The researchers can bring together methods which traditionally would have been an *"either/or"* option to better answer the question. He describes a feature of the mixed methods approach as having *"an explicit focus on the link between approaches, triangulation"* Ibid. He states that the mixed methods research is *"problem driven"* in that it is designed to answer the research problem as *"the over-riding concern"*.(Ibid).

3.4 Subjectivity and Bias

A qualitative study, even one that chooses to define itself within the broad family of 'mixed methods -can by its very definition be subjective and if, as is often the case, the researcher is working from a base of subject knowledge an ethical question of researcher bias arises. How much does the researcher`s own subject and experiential knowledge inform or direct the study? How much does the researcher`s own subject experience influence data content or gathering? Elliott et al (1999) acknowledges the subjectivity of the qualitative researcher and state "it *is impossible to put aside one's own perspectives totally"* but they advocate that the subject knowledge and values of the researcher *"can help to better understand represent the informants experiences more adequately than otherwise would have been possible"* ibid.

While planning and designing the study questions, I took the view that subjective background knowledge could be a positive element and would help to focus and inform the study design. There was an acute awareness of the importance of minimum intervention during the interviews. Research questions were designed to be open-ended and to guide topic discussion so that the respondent would talk about their experiences opinions and perceptions. Subjectivity therefore informed the design of the interviews as there was minimum intervention by the researcher during interviews. As the researcher, I had a very clear goal in data gathering to allow the data to speak for itself, and in that way, remove the implied bias of the researcher's background knowledge of the research topic. In more traditional research methodologies research assumptions could have been seen as *"bias and should be eliminated from the study"*. Rathith and Riggan (2012). This was the viewpoint taken by many early traditionalists. Post positivists have argued that subject knowledge is a bonus to the researcher rather than to be taken as *"an affliction, something to bear because it could not be foregone, could to the contrary be taken as to be virtuous"*. Glesne & Peshkin (1992, Pg. 104).

3.5 Needs Analysis

Rouda & Kusy (1995) define a needs assessment as "a systemic exploration of the way things are and the way things should be". Reviere et al describe an analysis of need as an analysis of "A gap between real and ideal that is both acknowledged by community values and potentially amenable to change" Reviere et al (1996). Widely used to assess a variation of consumer or project change, a needs assessment and analysis is often used in business or marketing circles to assess consumer needs in designing a product or service. Governments use a model of needs assessment to define the needs of any target community and much has been written about models of needs analysis. A paper written by U S government office of migrant education in 2001 to establish the educational needs of a migrant population outlined a 3 phase cycle as a "systemic approach that progresses through a defined series of phases ".

90

This template outlines the assessment and analysis process.

Explore "What is" Determine target groups	2 Gather and Analyse data Define needs	3 Prioritise needs Identify possible solutions

Table 3.1: Needs Analysis Template (US Gov 2001)

As part of this process, identifying major concerns and prioritising needs within the target group were seen as core to the establishment of the needs assessment and the identification of possible solutions.

"First you identify the audience and purposes for analysis, what McKillip 1998 calls the "users and uses" cited in Titcomb (2001). She describes the stages of identifying the stakeholders, their problems or needs which is followed by evaluation of the information collected from stakeholders to assist in the analysis of needs. Researchers in the field of education and training would typically use models of a Training Needs Analysis (TNA) to define, assess and analyse training needs of a programme to be delivered. Skillsnet writing in their Training Needs Analysis guide with regard to delivering training to business write that a good TNA would *"capture views of all stakeholders"* to identify problems and gaps in current training to identify stakeholder training needs. They recommend conducting surveys, interviews, focus groups, discussions within the population being studied as a means to gathering information.

Brown writing in his paper on needs assessment to define technical needs for a target population states that *"there is an expectation that action will follow the identification of disparities between the actual and the ideal"* Brown (2003). The needs analysis has an implied objective and is carried out on the basis that the needs of a population, group or community once identified which will lead to change or at the very least to recommendations for change to improve that community.

With its early roots in curriculum design, Ralph Tyler designed a model of needs analysis in 1949 which is still relevant today. Tyler's principles were:

6. state objectives,
7. select learning experiences,
8. organize learning experiences,
9. conduct evaluations Tyler, (1949).

Katz-Hass, an advocate of User Cantered Design models of information gathering and analysis suggests that a needs analysis defines the users or members of any group being analysed, in the mode of who? what ? and why? A User Centred Design model of a needs analysis project will identify the members of the group and what their functions and responsibilities are. It will examine their views and opinions on how their group or sector could function better. Katz-Haas (1998). Cavanagh and Chadwick writing on Health Needs Assessment describe a needs analysis as a review of issues facing a population *"leading to agreed priorities and resource allocation that will improve health and reduce inequalities"* NICE (2005). They describe a health needs analysis as being a flexible model to assess the needs of a particular population by gathering direct information and evaluation the priorities so that positive change is achieved.

The use of a needs analysis model to explore and evaluate the community of complementary therapies was considered the most appropriate method to identify the needs of that community. Through collecting and recording respondent experiences and opinions from within this target population, the study sought to learn about and identify gaps and possible solutions to the needs of this sector. Within the analysis, stakeholder roles, functions, individual views and opinions on how their own group should work were core to gathering information and identifying group concerns and needs and how these could be best addressed. Informed by the literature on needs analysis, the following model of assessment and analysis formed the basis of the study design.

1. Identify and contact CAM Stakeholders	2. Gather Direct Information Define concerns and needs	3 Prioritise Needs Make Recommendations for change

Table 3.2: Needs Analysis Sequence

3.6 Research Sampling Strategy

There are various methods of choosing samples to take part in online questionnaires. Medlin et al, describes three main categories of sampling an online population," *recruited samples, unrestricted and screened samples"* Medlin et al. (1999). A recruited sample is obtained by consulting directly with the intended sample and giving them direct access to the online survey with a web link, in the hope they will access the questionnaire and complete online. Unrestricted sampling is more general where a wider population is informed of the availability of an online questionnaire which anyone can access and complete. This was not the case for this particular study, as it was an aim of the research to recruit as many of the targeted sample as possible and as the sampling strategy was, as stated purposive, the sample was selected from CAM Learning Provider, Professional Association, Therapy Representatives and the Practitioner population.

In preparation for the survey efforts had been made to identify sector training providers and practitioner associations in several therapies, from available listings, who could be in a position to contribute to the survey. The sector is as described, a niche, specialist population and stakeholders involved in education, training and professional practice are a small population within that niche sector both in Ireland and within the EU. Within the context of this community stakeholders were identified and a sample was recruited according to purposive sampling strategy. Patton states that a purposeful or selective sampling is used by the researcher when in depth knowledge is considered to be rich and valuable to the study.and describes the strategy behind purposive sampling.

"The logic and power of purposeful sampling lies in selecting information-rich cases for study in depth. Information-rich cases are those from which one can learn a great deal from issues central to the purpose of the research, thus the term purposeful sampling, (Patton 1990,Pg.196).

It was considered that as many of the recruited sample had themselves established knowledge and experiences of their own sector that they could provide *"information rich."* data as described by Patton to inform the study.

The sample included the following categories.

- o Learning Providers across the diversity of CAM therapies.
- o Educators and Trainers within the CAM sector.
- o Representatives of CAM Professional Associations.
- o CAM representatives of UK and EU professional associations
- o Experienced CAM practitioners in several therapies.

Stakeholders had been selected from the following categories and had been included in the study as they had been identified and listed in a National Working Group Report to the Department for Health and Children (DOHC) report on the regulation of Complementary Therapists.

Categories as defined by the DOHC (Department of Health and Children) National Working Group Report on the Regulation of Complementary Therapists (2005)	
Category 1	Acupuncturists, Chiropractors, Homoeopaths, Osteopaths, Medical Herbalists
Category 2	Sports Therapists Massage therapists, Nutrition Therapists, Reflexologists, Aroma therapists, Reiki practitioners A range of CAM therapies being practiced in Ireland, listed in the next chapter.

Table 3.3: DOHC Categories for CAM Therapists

This report had categorised complementary therapists in terms of risk to the public, with category 1 therapies being considered a higher risk to the public than category 2. DOHC (2005). Within the contexts of risk to the public as described in this report, category 1 therapies defined their therapies as primary healthcare therapies with their own independent system of assessment, diagnosis and treatment. These are Acupuncture, Chinese Medicine, Homoeopathy, Herbalists. Chiropractors and Osteopaths although not participating directly in the DOHC consultation and working

95

group are typically considered to be of the same category and were included in the subsequent SMCI study commissioned by a joint DOHC and HETAC committee in 2010.SMCI (2012).

3.7 Purposive Sampling

Denscombe (2010) describes a purposive sample as *"handpicking"* a sample population deliberately to explore *"their privileged knowledge or experience about the topic"* (Pg. 35). He writes that purposive sampling works best with a known population when its knowledge and qualities are known to the researcher. He suggests that a purposive sample can be used as an exploratory exercise within a body of people when *" there are good grounds for believing they will be critical to the research"* Ibid. Using this sampling strategy the sample population are chosen on the basis of their *"relevance and knowledge"* of the topic being examined, Ibid.

The sample was taken from the wider CAM sector in Ireland where there is a variety of education, training and practice across the diversity of complementary therapies. Learning Providers in other countries with a similar structure were included in the sample to give a comparison of data to the study. Van Selms & Janowski (2006) describes the positive aspects of conducting online surveys, as the internet allows a researcher to identify potential respondents with the same background and interests, and make contact with them as potential participants in a web based project. One of the main reasons why the researcher employed a questionnaire is that it is now relatively easy to contact potential respondents via email. Robson,(2002),Bryman,(2008), write that delivering a questionnaire by internet communication, encourages a good response rate and is inexpensive for the researcher. All of the recruited respondents were known to be proficient with internet communication, as email correspondence was a regular and normal form of communication for the sample recruited.

An informational email explaining the purpose of the study and the survey, as part of a broader data collection strategy was sent to the pilot group, initially and then to the broader sample group. The email was motivational, explaining the ease of response, and the short period of time needed to complete the questionnaire. This was followed by another email with an embedded web link which would open the online questionnaire, when they clicked on the link. The direct link was used to make it easier for the potential respondents to complete the questionnaire

The following email requesting participation had been sent to potential respondents to canvas participation.

"Dear

The following survey is part of a broader study being conducted in Dublin City University on CAM Therapies.

As the study would benefit from as wide a response as possible from the CAM sector in Ireland, could you forward it to your members to complete, and also complete it yourself as Chair of the XX.

The survey link is embedded in this email and can be forwarded by email.

This is the direct link to the survey
http://www.surveymonkey.com/s/CAMDoctoralResearch

Analysis and publication will be published when the full study is complete in 2014. It is hoped that the information gathered in this survey and in the broader study will inform and benefit the CAM sector. Initial results being gathered suggest this information will be relevant to the sector.

Results will be made available to responders once published.

Thank you for your participation.

Kind Regards,

Bernadette Ward, MSc, PhD Candidate (2010-2014)"

3.8 Questionnaire Sample

250 stakeholders identified as representative of their therapy, were sent the email requesting participation, of which 172 responded in the full questionnaire sequence, which included the initial international pilot, a second Irish and EU pilot and a main questionnaire sent to Irish selected respondents.

172 significant CAM stakeholders in total participated in both the two pilot questionnaires and the main questionnaire, of which 10 international stakeholders completed the initial pilot questionnaire, which has been labelled Q1.

International respondents were CAM Learning Providers in Australia, Brazil, Canada, China, Malaysia, New Zealand South Africa, USA. All of those piloted had direct experience of CAM training, regulation, and practice in their own countries.

The 2nd pilot questionnaire was sent to 11 selected stakeholders in Ireland and the UK, of which 9 responded. This was labelled Q2. Early analysis of piloted questionnaire responses led to a reduction of questions in the main questionnaire. The rationale for this change is discussed in the following chapter on Data Collection, The main questionnaire, labelled Q3 was sent to a diversity of complementary therapists with roles in training, regulation and practice. Respondents represented more than 50 different therapies from all over Ireland.

3.8.1 Questionnaire Sequencing

172 Respondents

Q1	1st Pilot. Learning Providers International	10 respondents
Q2	2nd Pilot EU CAM stakeholders	9
Q3	CAM stakeholders, Learning Providers, Regulators, Practitioners	149
Q4	UK CAM Learning Providers	4

Table 3.4: Questionnaire Sequence

The following therapies represent the diversity of CAM therapies which are practiced in Ireland. Representatives of all of these therapies took part in the Q3 questionnaire.

Aromatherapy, Angelic Core Healing, Amatsu, Ayurveda, Bio-Energy, Bio Resonance, Bowen Technique,
Breathwork, Counselling Cranio-sacral Therapy, Dietetics, Ear Candling, Gua Sha, , Homoeopathy
Hypnotherapy, Kinesiology, Massage (Various) including, Deep tissue sports, Cancer care massage
Holistic, Indian Head Massage, Manual Lymphatic Drainage massage, Rebirthing, Remedial,
Seated Massage, Swedish Massage, Laser Therapy, Meditation, Meridian Therapy, Mindfulness,
Naturopathy, Neuromuscular Therapy, NLP Life Coaching, Psychotherapy, Quantum Touch, Qi Gong,
Reiki, Reflexology, Shen Therapy, Shiatsu, Sports, Stress Management,, Tai Chi,
Thermal Auricular Therapy, Visualisation, Yoga,

Table 3.5: Questionnaire Participant Categories

Questionnaire responses including respondent comments are discussed in the following chapter on Data Collection and Analysis.

3.9 Interview Sample - In depth Interviews

This initial questionnaire phase was followed by a 2nd phase of 20 qualitative in depth semi structured interviews of selected CAM stakeholders. Stakeholders were selected on the basis that they were experienced learning providers, were involved with professional regulation or had significant experience within the this sector. It was considered that some complementary therapy professionals who were active and were the product of some of the training programmes delivered in Ireland and in other countries for the purposes of comparative analysis should be included in the study as their experiences were considered relevant to the study. Interviews are commonly used as a second sequence within a study framework and are a customary qualitative research tool.

Semi structured interviews give more *"flexibility of response"* to both the interviewer and the interviewee according to Robson. Depth interviews allow the respondent to say whatever they like about the subject, without intervention from the interviewer and only *"minimum prompting"*, Robson (2007 Pg. 270).

The majority of interviews were conducted with Irish CAM stakeholders, however, non-Irish interviews were also conducted to give a reference of comparison to the sector in Ireland. One to one interviews were conducted with UK participants and with broader EU and international participants. All recordings were transcribed verbatim, in as far as possible. The list of interview participants are outlined in the following table.

3.9.1 Interview Participants

Interview participants are listed by initials, numbers and role within the CAM sector. The table of participants is on the following page in table 3.6.

Participant	Role	Country
1 AM	Learning Provider	Ireland
2 AV	Regulator/Practitioner	Ireland
3 HB	Learning Provider/Practitioner	Ireland
4 CC	Trainer/Practitioner	Ireland
5 DM	Regulator/Practitioner	Ireland
6 LM	Regulator/Practitioner	Ireland
7 GM	Learning Provider	Ireland
8 AM	Learning Provider	Ireland
9 MR	Learning Provider	Ireland
10 CR	Regulator/Practitioner	Ireland
11 DS	Learning Provider/Practitioner	Ireland
12 CO	Regulator/Practitioner	Ireland
13 JW	Teacher/Practitioner	UK
14 FM	Regulator/Teacher	UK
15 TP	Teacher/Practitioner	UK
16 SB	Teacher/Practitioner	UK
17 AH	Regulator/Practitioner	UK
18 DZ	Regulator/Teacher	Holland
19 RD	Learning Provider	Spain
20 RB	Learning Provider	Brazil

Table 3.6: List of Interview Participants

Interview planning, and data collected from the one to one interviews are discussed in a following chapter on Data Collection and Analysis.

3.10 Study Triangulation

Triangulation within a single study is often used as a method of verification of study results, and is typically used in social sciences research. Adami & Kiger (2005) described it as the use of more than one and sometimes *"multiple methods for gathering and/ or handling data within a single study"* with the original purpose being *"to seek confirmation of apparent findings"*. They suggest that there is now support for the use of triangulation to give *"completeness* "to a study. Quantitative research can provide positivist data which can validate a study whereas qualitative data can seek to address the inquiry explorative aspect of a study. Using two or more methods within a single study with a single researcher can help to address perceived bias for qualitative research, and help to strengthen study validity. The concept of triangulation, borrowed from the world of surveying, according to Punch (2010 when a method of triangulation is used to answer the research question it *"enhances confidence in the ensuing findings"* Denzin (1978) describes several ways that triangulation can be used within a study either to gather or analyse data. He describes his theories and listed the different type of triangulation as to include data, investigator or researcher, theory or methodological. His descriptions are listed as follows.

- Data triangulation: involves time, space, and persons
- Investigator triangulation: involves multiple researchers in an investigation
- Theory triangulation: involves using more than one theoretical scheme in the interpretation of the phenomenon
- Methodological triangulation: involves using more than one method to gather data, such as interviews, observations, questionnaires, and documents.

He identified "*Methodological Triangulation*" as using more than one method of study such as questionnaires, interviews, observations and documents. This is the most frequent method of triangulation. Webb et al. (1966), wrote that a hypothesis or proposition which is *"confirmed by two or more independent measurement processes, the uncertainty of its interpretation is greatly reduced"*. Bryman (2007) writes that triangulation is useful within a research study *"in terms of adding a sense of richness and complexity to the enquiry"*. He writes that using triangulation can add confidence to the study findings. This study has used methodological triangulation as described by Denzin, by using two different methodologies to research the same subject and address the same research problem. Analysis of the different methodologies to answer the same research questions is intended to strengthen validity of the research

103

methodologies. The use of both gave the researcher the opportunity to verify both datasets with each other, which strengthened study findings.

3.11 Study Generalisation

The ability to generalise data collected in any study is a goal for researchers. Polit & Beck describe generalisation as *"an act of reasoning that draws broad inferences from particular observations"* They write that quantitative researchers would use generalisation as a research standard but it is not as common within qualitative research. Firestone (1993) wrote about three types of generalisation, statistical generalisation, mostly used in quantitative research *"from a sample to a population."* Analytical generalisation, which according to Polit & Beck has relevance in both quantitative and quantitative research. They also describe Firestones third type of generalisation as *"case to case generalisation"* often described as transferability and mostly used in case studies. Positivist quantitative research traditions using quantitative research tools such as surveys clearly have explicit generalisation acceptance within the wider scientific community. Social researchers using post positivist research methods in empirical research studies need to plan and design the study so that generalisation of study data is considered.

Williams (2000) advocates *Moderatum Generalization* as being a social researcher's aspiration using qualitative research methods. Qualitative research findings can have a moderate generalisation function rather than sweeping generalisations from the study to the universe. These generalisations like any other within the research communities will hold until further research findings can produce evidence, whether achieved through positivist or post positivist, even interpretivist studies challenge or add clarification to findings. Generalisation within this study has been considered in the planning and design of the study within the niche population being studied in this research. Context of this study is the CAM educational and professional practice sector and data collected from within this sector should help to inform the wider CAM population policy makers.

David Peters (BMJ 2013) writing in the British Medical Journal discusses *"implementation research"* within the health service in which a niche study can be carried out in a small or pilot population with the intention of wider application across the health service.

He discusses implementation research as being focused on *"the users of research"* such as particular stakeholders within a population or service, rather than adding to the broader research knowledge.

> *"Context plays a central role in implementation research. Context can include the social, cultural, economic, political, legal, and physical environment, as well as the institutional setting, comprising various stakeholders and their interactions, and the demographic and epidemiological conditions, ibid.*

Context within the study is relevant to study planning and design and potential generalisation of study findings within the communities being researched, both within the national context and the wider CAM communities.

3.11.1 Study Ethics Approval

Prior to the study commencement, I received ethics approval from the DCU ethics committee in accordance with the guidelines of this university. As all participants of the study are adult volunteers, this was considered by the university to be a low risk study. In line with the university's Plain Language Statement requirements, all participants were provided with details of the study, including working title, purpose and aims of the study. They were informed that as volunteers, they could withdraw any time they wished. They were given details of their involvement with the study, including details of how interviews, would be conducted and recordings and transcriptions made with their agreement. They were informed they could request a copy of their interview transcript and make any changes they were not happy with. There were no perceived risks to participants and they were assured of confidentiality. They were advised that the intention of the study was to provide information to the CAM sector and it was hoped that participants may benefit indirectly from the study findings. They were assured that the researcher would make every effort to respect their anonymity and that all notes, transcripts and records would be stored in a secure location.

Conclusion

This chapter described the mythological paradigm of the study, describing the post positivist framework which guided the study. It confirmed that the study received ethics approval from the university ethics committee. It explained how the study evolved to become a broader needs analysis of the CAM sector. This chapter discussed purposive sampling and outlined the study sampling strategy and recruitment for both the quantitative and qualitative elements of the study, describing the rationale of participant selection. It discussed the background and the literature on models of needs analysis of target communities. Finally this chapter discussed how study triangulation and generalisation were included within study design and planning together with a discussion on how subjectivity and bias was addressed within the study.

Chapter 4 Data Collection and Analysis

4.1 Introduction

This Chapter outlines the collection of data from both the questionnaire and the in depth interviews. It discusses the rationale for the use of a mixed methods online questionnaire and details the process of data collection, from both the questionnaire and the interviews. Design and planning of questions and the inclusion of comment text boxes within the questionnaire are outlined and explained. Data collection sequence is outlined and explained. Interviews with selected stakeholders was described in terms of method and venue. The rationale of using a flexible paradigm within the interview strategy in order to allow a wider discussion of the topic was described. Data analysis methodology for both the quantitative and qualitative data was discussed in relation to summative data for the quantitative elements and the use of a thematic coding framework for analysing the qualitative data.

4.2 Data Collection Sequence

Phase 1	Phase 2	Phase 3
Quantitative Online Survey	Survey Comment Boxes (Qualitative)	In Depth Stakeholder Interviews

Table 4.1: Data Collection Sequence

The sequencing of research methods used was chosen to use the quantitative survey in the initial phase to provide base study data followed by the qualitative in depth interviews to expand the data and to delve further into the research subject. Punch(2010) states that both quantitative and qualitative methods share many similarities from a basis of different approaches. Quantitative is *"more concerned with the deductive testing of hypotheses and theories"* It approaches the study from knowledge of possible outcomes and will typically collect data to measure and test the theory. Qualitative is more concerned with inductively exploring a hypothesis or theory and *although it is the most favoured approach for generating theory it can also test hypothesis and theories"*, Punch (2010 Pg. 235). Miles and Huberman say that *"both types of data can be productive for descriptive, reconnoitring, exploratory, inductive, opening up purposes"*,(1994 Pg.42).

4.2.1 Data Collection Questionnaire

The questionnaire, which was piloted, focused on stakeholder role, details of various aspects of the provision of CAM training, including whether respondents had achieved academic validation or professional accreditation of courses. Obstacles to training and practice, regulation status, public expectations and sector needs were all included within the pilot questionnaire. Survey Monkey software permits the building of a respondent email database, which can initially be used to deliver the questionnaire and later can be used to send reminders to those whom the software has identified as non- responders. It allows flexibility in the preparation of questions, the tracking of survey responses and the ability to add to or change wording or focus of questions. The use of the programme to record all responses on a hard drive on a remote server adds a number of useful functions in the collection and recording of data, on a web based database which can be accessed on demand by the researcher.

"The WWW software program prepares the questionnaire file and stores it on the internet hard drive so it is ready to generate computer screens for completion by each respondent. Instead of responses being recorded on paper they are stored on a secure hard disk drive at a remote internet site", Medlin et al (1999).

Dilman et al (1999) discusses the necessity to design `respondent-friendly` survey design, making it easy for the respondent to understand what is being asked, with clear instructions as to how to respond so as *"to decrease the occurrence of measurement and non-response errors in surveys"* Pg..3. Under the definition of respondent-friendly survey design Dilman writes about aspects of *"access, motivation and cognition"*, Ibid.

Potential respondents must be able to easily access the questionnaire, or be able to complete it online, on a variation of web browsers and devices, which are in common use today.

> *"They must be able to comprehend what is expected of them, know what actions are required for responding and be motivated to take those actions"*, Ibid.

Questions were built using a combination of fixed design multiple choice responses on a click and go basis, while adding text boxes where relevant and encouraging open ended responses. The online survey tool used for this study was, as stated, Survey Monkey, an interactive, easy to use survey tool with the possibility of designing a range of question types which would permit using both quantitative and qualitative question types. The survey can be sent in an email to a selected sample with easy to open web links. It is designed to collect all responses and is easy for the respondents to use and complete. Explanations for each question can be inserted so that the respondent has a clear idea of the purpose of the question. According to Robson,

> *"surveys are almost always carried out as part of a non-experimental fixed design which can be used for any research purposes, whether exploratory, descriptive, explanatory or emancipatory"*, Ibid (Pg. 232).

Both quantitative and qualitative elements within the questionnaire were intended to address the fixed and explorative aspects of the research questions. Bryman (2007) supported the use of both quantitative and qualitative methodologies together in a study

109

design. The researcher had previous experience in using Survey Monkey software. Online questionnaires have become a regular tool for the researcher in all sectors, and the design of the questionnaire cannot emulate a traditional paper questionnaire. Sheehan and McMillan (1999) suggest that conventional postal type surveys with several pages are not a suitable online survey and can negatively affect the response rate. Survey design is crucial to response rates and questions should be clear and in plain language with the principle of short clear questions in an accessible questionnaire. Online survey response rates have demonstrated that the longer the questionnaire, the less likely people will respond, Dillman et al. (1998). Respondents to email and online surveys are also more willing to complete text boxes and respond to open ended questions, giving a qualitative, post positivist aspect to a mixed method survey then they would be to conventional fixed question questionnaires. The questionnaire contained both closed and open ended questions. In a review of three email surveys Sheehan and McMillan (1999) found that respondents seemed to be much more willing to reply to open-ended questions in an email format than in traditional paper survey style questionnaires.

4.2.2 Survey Comment Boxes

Comment boxes added to several relevant questions included the words *"Please feel free to discuss in the comment box"*. This was intended in the post positivist style of enquiry to permit expansion on responses and generate more in-depth data than the quantitative responses permitted. I had intended that the addition of comment boxes would allow respondents to expand on some of the short question responses, so there would be an element of the respondents own words within the survey. Completion of the comment boxes was not mandatory, respondents could choose whether to expand on their responses or not. Each question required a response before the respondent could progress to the next question. Bryman (1988) advocates that the use of both quantitative and qualitative elements within a survey or questionnaire can provide richer data for the researcher. He suggests that using both methods would compensate for any weakness in either methodology and would *"capitalise on the strengths of the two approaches.* The questionnaire (Q1), was piloted by first sending to a group of CAM stakeholders, who had been selected from an international listing. This was intended, not only to test the questionnaire delivery and response, but to gather base data from other countries, which could be considered as comparative information for the study.

Questions included in the initial pilot questionnaire are outlined in the following table.

1	Describe courses in Complementary Medicine you are familiar with.
2	Please discuss briefly the legal status of Complementary Medicine in your country?
3	Are courses you are familiar with privately operated?
4	How is professional practice of your therapy or therapies if more than one regulated in Ireland?
5	Have any courses in your therapy achieved academic validation of their courses at any level?
6	Please explain what changes, if any were necessary in preparation for academic validation of your course?
7	Are courses in your therapy accredited by the professional associations?
8	Please discuss Quality Assurance Procedures in relation to your course?
9	Do patients who seek treatments ask about regulation or registration of the practitioner??
10	Are patients aware of the differences between Professional accreditation and Academic validation of CAM courses relevant to the practitioner's training?
11	Should there be a model of national regulation and registration of practitioners in Ireland?

Table 4.2: Q1 Questionnaire Questions

In consideration of the study's flexible paradigm, pilot survey responses were analysed early and some changes were made to the survey, based on the responses. Initial analysis of the first survey responses suggested that small changes would be made to the questions to provide clarification before it was out to a wider population.

The following questions were added to the questionnaire.

List the therapy or therapies if more than one that you work with? Choose one of the following to best represent the area you work with 1. Learning Provider 2. Regulation. 3 Teacher   4 Practice
HETAC and FETAC prior to their merger into QQI recently removed the academic awards standard for Complementary Therapies in Ireland so currently there is no route to academic validation of courses at any level of the National qualifications framework.
Should the newly formed QQI restore the CAM academic awards standard and include CAM courses in the National Framework of Qualification Awards?

Table 4.3: Additional Questions for Main Questionnaire

A second pilot questionnaire was sent to a selected group of stakeholders in Ireland and the UK who were known to be active in their communities.

Early analysis of the first two pilot questionnaires, with regard to the focus and relevance of all of the questions, and ease of respondent completion, as discussed, led to a decision to reduce the number of questions for the subsequent main questionnaire. Findings from Q1 and Q2 demonstrated that topics could be summarised within the questionnaire, as some of the questions had addressed different aspects of the same topic such as quality assurance, and validation. The researcher also believed that the questionnaire could be improved with, fewer more focused questions. It was decided to continue with text comment boxes and encourage respondents to add their opinions and views. A shorter, more focused questionnaire was regarded as easier for the respondents and would encourage wider completion of the questionnaire. Question focus remained linked to aspects of the research questions , which Q1 and Q2 had addressed.

Subsequently the questionnaire (Q3) was sent to a wider sample of CAM stakeholders. The following questionnaire with a reduced number of 13 questions, was sent to a wider CAM sample reflecting several therapies and stakeholders. Brief explanations were given for each question within the questionnaire. More comment boxes were added and respondents were encouraged to add their comments in the vein of *"Please expand on your response*, or *"Please add your comments* " The literature had been acknowledged as previously stated by Dillman et al (1998) that shorter questionnaires are more appropriate for online use and demonstrate a better response rate. Of the 250 CAM stakeholders who had been sent emails requesting their participation 149 stakeholders responded and completed the Q 3 questionnaire. Reminders had been sent to those who did not initially respond, and that did provide a further small number of responses. Responses demonstrated that the majority of people who clicked on the email link completed the questionnaire. It had been hoped that the use of comment boxes would provide "raw data" from the respondents which the closed questions could not provide. Respondents did add their comments on several topics, which gave the researcher some further information on the topics being explored, and did provide some rich data on respondent opinions and viewpoints.

Q3 questions and question information are outlined in the table in the following page.

Q 3 question information and questions.

1.Identification of CAM Therapies List the therapy or therapies if more than one that you work with?
2.Choose one of the following to best represent the area you work with Professional Association, Training, Practice.
3. Evidence of Effect: Is there published evidence of effect for any of the therapies you are associated with?
4. Professional Regulation; How is professional practice of your therapy or therapies if more than one regulated in Ireland?
5. Professional Associations; Is there is more than 1 professional association for your therapy
6. Professional Standards. If there is more than 1 professional association for your therapy do any of the following options apply? There is broad national agreement on standards of practitioner training between the associations?
7. Education and Training; Are there more than 1 training courses for your therapy in Ireland
8. How are CAM courses delivered?
9. Professional Accreditation; Are courses in your therapy professionally accredited?
10. Academic Validation of Courses; Have any courses in your therapy achieved academic validation of their courses at any level?
11. Public Awareness Do patients who seek treatments ask about regulation or registration of the practitioner?
12. Are patients aware of the differences between Professional accreditation and Academic validation of CAM courses relevant to the practitioner's training?
13. Future of CAM in Ireland Should there be a model of national regulation and registration of practitioners?

Table 4.4: Q3 Questions From Online Questionnaire.

4.3 Data Collection Interviews

This initial phase was followed by a 2nd phase of 20 qualitative in depth semi structured interviews of selected CAM stakeholders. Interviews are commonly used as a second sequence within a study framework and are a customary qualitative research tool. An open ended semi structured question guide based on the research questions was prepared for possible interviewees. Relevant stakeholders were contacted by email, outlining the study objectives and requesting participation. Semi structured interviews give more *"flexibility of response"* to both the interviewer and the interviewee according to Robson. Early analysis of some of the questionnaire results informed the design of the guide questions, which were used in the interviews. Ribbins and Marland (1994) write about preparing an agreed interview schedule in the preparation of guide questions which are then sent to possible interviewees. They describe their interviews as *"discussions"* or *"conversations "*, rather than adopting the interviews as an exercise in delivering questions and receiving answers. They also discuss an aspect of flexibility as the interviews or discussions continue.

They suggest that

> *"An advantage over the interview-based approach is that it is possible to revise and renegotiate the agenda of discussion as a natural aspect of the dialogue" ,(Pg. 7).*

Punch (2010) discusses theoretical generation as part of data collection, in that in the early interviews a theory may emerge which may not have been part of the guide questions, so can be included in subsequent interviews. Informal first data analysis is taking place as the data is being collected. This adds to and influences further data collection. Glaser and Strauss (1967) states that grounded theory is faithful to its philosophical roots in pragmatism.

Punch described a route from researcher questions to final data analysis Punch (2010 Pg.158). The following outline reflects the ongoing early analysis of data throughout data collection.

Data Collection 1	Data Analysis 1
Data Collection 2	Data Analysis 2
Data Collection 3	Data Analysis 3

Table 4.5: Table Data Analysis Sequence (Punch 2010)

As the interview continues and the respondent opinions and experiences are relayed, additional questions can be added if the respondent is enlarging on a particular subject. The researcher was mindful of the research questions and the focus of the study, but in some case the respondent was encouraged to further explain an event or opinion, expanding on the question guide. Depth interviews allow the respondent to say whatever they like about the subject, without intervention from the interviewer with only *"minimum prompting"*. Robson (2007, Pg. 270).

4.3.1 Interview Process

One to one interviews, arranged by appointment with the interviewee, can often form a useful part of a mixed method research study. My goal in conducting the interviews was to encourage the respondent to discuss the topic and let the data collected in the interviews speak for itself, without interruption or interference. Appointments were made with 20 stakeholders, representing an estimated 70% of the CAM community in Ireland, and face to face or Skype interviews were arranged. Gibson and Brown (2009) state that *"New communicative modes of web based communication have dramatically enhanced the range of media through which interviews can be conducted"* ,(Pg. 93). They suggest that using the telephone or other media can be more convenient for both the researcher and the respondent. The interviews took place by pre arrangement with stakeholders who had received an initial e-mail, informing them of the study and asking for their participation in

116

a one to one interview. Once a positive response was received from the participant, they were telephoned to make the specific arrangements and to answer any questions the interviewee may have and to confirm venue, date and time. Most of the selected interviewees were available to meet face-to-face and agreed to the interview recorded, however four of the interviewees were not easily available to meet face to face and agreed to Skype interviews. I subsequently organised a Skype account with a facility to telephone respondents on either their mobile or landline numbers and record their interviews. Familiarity with Skype was not necessary as my Skype account was sufficient to make contact with participants at the phone number they chose. Skype was chosen because it was considered the most reliable method of recording telephone interviews. I had previously downloaded a specific MP3 recorder, which integrates with the Skype software and records telephone interviews, which are then retained in an MP3 file for later transcription. Some interviewees had requested the guide questions before the interview and in those cases, they were emailed to them, but during the interview there was no intervention by the researcher, except occasional prompts if there interviewee was veering away from the subject. I felt that once the interviewee relaxed, they spoke openly and some at length, on subjects which interested them, or they had particular experience in. Many of them they spoke with passion about the work and experiences they had spent adult lives involved in. Silverman discusses representing the experiences of the interviewee, within the context of those experiences *"The primary issue is to generate data which give an authentic insight into people`s experiences"* Silverman,(2001) cited in Silverman (2011 Pg. 133). He discusses the necessity of attributing *"the meanings people attribute to their* social *world"* Ibid, so that the researcher can gain knowledge from the interview, beyond the words of the interviewee, as he advocates that the meanings and contexts are all relevant to the post positivist interviewer

Venues were chosen to suit the interviewee and I encouraged the interviewee to choose a quiet venue where the interviewee could speak freely. Denscombe writes about arranging an interview venue *"with fairly good acoustics and some measure of privacy "*(Pg. 182)

117

and he also suggests that seating arrangements, eye contact, comfort of the interviewee should be considered. He advocates setting up the seating arrangements so that there is good *"Interaction between the researcher and interviewee"* Ibid. While a choice of quiet venue which offered some privacy was suggested to the potential respondents on the telephone, the choice of venue was in most cases suggested by the interviewee. The majority of interviews were conducted with Irish CAM stakeholders, however, non-Irish interviews were also conducted to provide a comparison to the sector in Ireland. One to one interviews were conducted with UK participants and with broader EU and international participants.

The study used a flexible design so the data was continuously revisited during data collection so that early data could be analysed initially to inform further data collection. According to Robson

> *"In flexible designs there should be repeated revisiting of all of the aspects as the research takes place. In other words the detailed framework of the design emerges during the study",* Robson *(2009,Pg. 81).*

This was especially relevant in early interviews as respondents discussed and expanded on guide topics and in some cases added additional topics. In those cases I made no effort to stop or redirect the interviewee, especially if an emerging topic was interesting and has some relevance to the overall study. I encouraged further discussion and asked them to expand on the topic on the occasions when that occurred during the interview. The Glaser and Strauss (1967) grounded theory concept is based on the principles that theory emerges from the data as the research is being evaluated as it emerges through constant comparison of events or concepts.

Strauss and Corbin (1978) write that

> *"theory evolves during actual research and it does this by continuous interplay between data gathering and analysis",(Pg. 274).*

As the interviews were semi-structured there was the flexibility to allow new concepts to emerge from the data. Some of the interviewees were experienced learning providers and I wished to take the opportunity to ask about course validation and accreditation, professional regulation, course governance and funding. I canvassed their experiences and opinions on operating within the current vacuum of regulation and guidance, and whether this impacted or limited their work. I also sought their opinions on the need for quality oversight of both training and practice and the views on how this could be provided. Those topics were relevant to practitioners who were also regulators as they had undertaken CAM courses and had direct experience in that area. Interviewees were asked to comment on public demand and attitudes to their therapies in terms of access, safety and regulation. They were asked to discuss any issues they had, and what their concerns for the sector were. Interviewees were encouraged to discuss any aspect of their work and life as part of this sector which they considered important. Finally they were asked for their opinions on what their future plans were and what they thought the CAM sector needed to progress.

Several of them spoke about their personal investment in their work both in terms of time personal and financial effort, far beyond what could be expected from more main stream work. This has not been considered by me in designing the topic questions and was added to the guide question list for further interviews. Another theme which began to emerge from some of the early interviews, which had been listed as a discussion topic in the guide questions was the significance of personal and job satisfaction that some of the interviewees referred to. This too was then added to the list of guide topics for further interviewees, as those who spoke about it did so with strong emphasis or passion.

4.3.2 Data Preparation

Interview recordings, as stated, were typed, in most cases soon after the recordings, to provide transcripts for analysis. For some of the later interviews I used "Dragon Speech to Text" software to transcribe the interviews. A system of ongoing editing of the text to correct any inaccuracies was found to be an efficient and effective way to transcribe the data. It also provided me with the opportunity to become immersed in the data and to once again become very familiar with the interviews as well as the text generated from the text comment boxes. Respondents were informed they could request a transcript of their interview for verification if they wished. The transcriptions were by intent verbatim, so that the data transcribed was faithful to the data collected and the respondents own words. All interviewees and survey participants were informed that they could have access to study results on completion, following submission to the university, and completion of the study.

While the quantitative survey questions in the first sequence of data collection could provide the factual data to answer some of these questions, stakeholder experiences, opinions, future plans could only be explored within the qualitative in depth stakeholder interviews and survey comment boxes provided for some of the questions. According to Dawson *"Qualitative research explores attitudes, behaviours and experiences in an attempt to get an in depth opinion from participants"* so interviews were chosen as the main qualitative element in the study to delve into the direct experiences and opinions of the stakeholders, and the therapies many of them represented, selected for this study, Dawson (2009 Pg. 14). Ribbins and Marland observe that although the interviewer can gain a lot of information from the interviewee, it is more productive to let them talk and *"They will say a good deal more about themselves"*, Ibid. This was the approach that I adopted in preparing and conducting the semi structured interviews. Stakeholders interviewed were, as stated, selected on the basis of their experience and knowledge of working in this sector and their roles in the representation of their therapies. Denscombe (2010), writes about selecting subjects for research who are in the best position to provide the information that the researcher is seeking. He discusses target and selection sampling and describes purposive sampling as being

> *"about getting the best information by selecting items or people or people most likely to have the experience or expertise to provide quality and valuable insights on the research topic".(Pg. 35).*

120

4.4 Data Analysis Methodology

Green (2007) described mixed methods data analysis and analytical strategies as *"importantly connected to but not dictated by prior methodological decisions "* (Pg. 143). Although the researcher in choosing a mixed methodology *"indicates broad analytical directions, but rarely specifies particular procedures or strategies"*, Ibid. Greene suggests that in the *"component stage"*, (Pg. 144) of data collection , both methods can continue independently of each other, and it can be at the analysis or findings stages that the integration or linking of both methods takes place. As this study, as stated was sequential with the quantitative element of the questionnaire providing base, demographic, and sector foundation information which informed the study, and provided "what" of the research questions, and the qualitative element provided the broader informational data, both methods were inter dependent and connected, although not linked at the data collection or analysis stages. Both methods were complementary and collaborative and in combination were intended to *"provide a cohesive and singular understanding of the problem being investigated"*, Johnson & Onwuegbuzie, (2004). This Chapter discusses how both data sets are analysed separately, although both answering different aspects of the same study questions, and will outline how the findings are linked, within a thematic coding framework.

4.4.1 Quantitative Questionnaire Data

Robson (2002) discusses different methods of analysing quantitative data, as data sets broadly fall into two categories, exploratory and the confirmatory.

> *"Exploratory analysis explores the Data, trying to find out what it can tell you and confirmatory analysis seeks to establish whether you have actually got which are expected", (Pg. 399).*

He describes EDA (exploratory data analysis) which modern researchers have used within the quantitative framework, to explain findings that were not expected or confirmed expectations from quantitative data responses.

As part of the mixed methods, exploratory paradigms both quantitative and qualitative analysis was used. The study, as stated, worked within what is primarily an exploratory framework. However, when analysing data from responses to questions collected from the online survey, both exploratory and confirmatory analysis was used where relevant. Responses to the closed positivist questions could be considered to be confirmatory analysis. For example, it is already known within the Irish community that most CAM learning providers are private institutions as the majority of courses are delivered privately. Nevertheless it was necessary to establish this within the context of a question within the survey therefore the response was confirmatory of expectations. Response results for this question, as expected, confirmed that most courses in complementary therapies are provided by private learning providers, whether that is an individual or a group of individuals.

The survey monkey software has the capacity to analyse question responses in terms of frequency analysis, and percentages and will allow the researcher to work with the recorded data, prioritising and comparing responses. Individual questionnaires using a combination of closed and open ended questions are collated by the software. Responses can be organised and summarised within the software functionality so that results of each question can be presented in various formats. Closed question responses can be quantified in numeric terms, such as percentages, and ratios, both in individual responses which are then organised and collated collectively, question by question in the survey report provided by the analysis software. Open ended question responses are gathered and retained on an individual basis as well as being organised and collated to produce a collective report showing all open ended responses. Emergent themes derived from the open ended questions were categorised in relation to the main aspects of the research questions so the questionnaire could be analysed using a mix of methods. It was at first planned to retain qualitative data from comment box content for later analysis with the main body of qualitative data derived from interview transcripts, however I considered that because the open ended responses and comment boxes formed an integral part of the questionnaire, they should be analysed alongside the survey responses. Emergent and recurring themes from the text derived from both the open ended responses and text box comments and opinions were categorised according to the study qualitative analysis framework, and each theme given a value for ease of analysis, within the concept of content analysis. These categories are set out in the following paragraph.

Although the survey software has the capacity to analyse qualitative text, it was decided to handle all qualitative text within an Excel based thematic coding framework, using frequency and comparative analysis to record emerging themes and concepts.

"A simple means of exploring many data sets used to recast them in a way which counts the frequency that certain things happen, or to find ways of displaying that information. So frequency analysis and a comparative analysis will help to develop dominant themes within qualitative analysis and coding", Robson (2002 Pg. 403).

Denscombe (2010) discusses working with the raw data in terms of

"organising, summarising and displaying the evidence and describing the findings", (Pg. 241).

He writes about "exploring connections between parts of the data correlations and associations", Ibid.

The researcher used a combination of survey monkey's own analytical tools and Excel spreadsheets to analyse data collected from the questionnaire.

The following is a screenshot of one of analysis of one of the survey questions (www.surveymonkey.com)

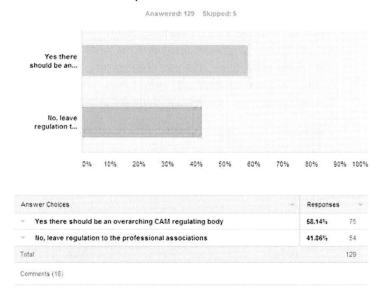

Future of CAM in Ireland Should there be a model of national regulation and registration of practitioners in Ireland

Answered: 129   Skipped: 5

Answer Choices		Responses	
▾ Yes there should be an overarching CAM regulating body		58.14%	75
▾ No, leave regulation to the professional associations		41.86%	54
Total			129

Comments (16)

Figure 4.1: Surveymonkey.com Example of Question Analysis

The following 2nd Screenshot is a collection of respondent comments gathered by Survey Monkey in the analysis of a survey question.

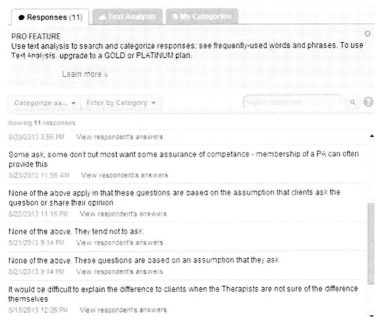

Figure 4.2: Surveymonkey.com Example of Questionnaire Comments

4.4.2 Qualitative Data Analysis Transcripts

A content thematic analysis framework was used where the qualitative data in text format was examined for emerging themes. Qualitative data was examined and read through by the researcher several times in order to identify recurring themes and so the researcher became very familiar with the data. In discussing thematic analysis and as Silverman 2011 suggests the researchers should *"familiarise themselves with their data set"*, so that initial themes could be labelled or coded, and in that way *"systematically code the whole dataset "* (Pg. 274). In that process he suggests the researcher searches for themes, refine them and generate a *"thematic map diagram"* Ibid. An inductive approach of raw data analysis was systemically used so that themes emerging from the data were categorised into labels or codes. Raw data produced from both the survey comment boxes and interview transcripts were

125

organised to define a frame using an inductive approach of thematic analysis. Themes were grouped to examine frequencies and similarities of codes emerging from the data. Dawson (2009), describes the inductive approach as *"themes emerging from the data and not imposed upon it"* (Pg. 119). It was always my intention to allow themes to emerge organically from the raw data, so this approach was considered to be the best fit. Comparative analysis was also used to compare responses from different respondents. *"Closely connected to thematic analysis is comparative analysis"* ibid. Comparative analysis of emergent themes from data derived from different people within the sample and this continues during analysis of the full sample until the researcher is satisfied that no new themes are emerging.

In preparation for defining an analytical coding frame data is read several times, and "cleaned" to isolate data which is not relevant to the research study. According to Pope, Zibland and Mays (2000) *"immersion in the data is an important first step in analysis"*. Interview transcripts were read initially without applying any thematic codes. Reading the data initially without coding *"to identify emergent themes without losing the connections between concepts and context"*(ibid) is an effective method of early data analysis. Only after becoming familiar with the content did I begin initial open coding of the texts, applying labels to the emerging themes. Codes according to Miles and Huberman (1994) are tags or labels which are categorised on sentences or groups of words within the data which describe the experiences of the subjects. Labels are used to identify recurring themes within the data in terms of relevance to the research questions and research objectives. This gives a systemic structure to the analysis of the research data. Morse advocates that a single researcher is the preferred choice for identifying themes and defining codes, Morse (1999). Initial codes formed the frame for data content analysis for later interviews. Gibson and Brown (2009) advocate that Apriori codes relating to the study questions and interest and empirical codes which can evolve interactively from within the data can help define data codes. They suggest that while *"some Apriori categories may be specified in advance of the analysis of date, most codes will be defined interactively"*, (ibid Pg..135).

In the initial stages of data examination, thematic codes were applied by highlighting text within the word document and adding labels within comment boxes. A decision was taken to use Microsoft Excel to organise data codes and thematic labels. This was chosen in preference to some of the qualitative analysis software such as NVIVO due to familiarity with Excel and a preference to be more in immersed within data labelling. Sidebars of interesting and relevant text from respondent's transcriptions were added to the summery. Respondents were asked to talk about their own experiences as CAM stakeholders.

The following Screenshot is an example of thematic coding of interviews,

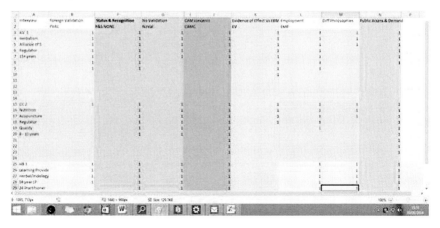

Figure 4.3: Example of Qualitative Thematic Coding
Recurring themes from those responses were labelled according to relevance to the research questions and also to the frequency of emergent themes.

Both methods of data collection and analysis were by intent complementary and collaborative. In linking both Quantitative and Qualitative Findings, the following table outlines which aspects of the study question was addressed by the quantitative findings and which aspects were addressed by the Qualitative findings. Some

127

parts of the study problem were addressed by both the quantitative and qualitative. These are outlined in a table in Chapter 5.

Conclusion

This chapter outlined the collection of both the quantitative and qualitative data. It described the quantitative data collection process and detailed the questionnaire sequencing, from the initial pilot to the wider study sample. It described how the pilot questionnaire informed the preparation of the main questionnaire and some questions were changed following early analysis of piloted responses. In depth interview preparation and process was discussed, using minimum intervention by the researcher to allow broader data to emerge from the interviews. The rationale of allowing new guide topics to emerge from early interviews to be added to later interviews was described. The philosophy and methodology used for data analysis for both the quantitative and qualitative data was discussed. The qualitative data analysis methodology, using a thematic framework for recurring and comparative themes throughout the text data was described.

Chapter 5 Results and Findings

5.1 Introduction

In the following chapter, themes which emerged both from the qualitative and qualitative elements of this study are outlined, and discussed. Quantitative results from questionnaire data is presented in the format of percentages in chart and diagram format. Dominant themes which emerged from qualitative data are presented, representing questionnaire respondent comments within the text boxes and stakeholder interview transcripts. Six main themes emerged from the raw qualitative data, which had been identified, on analysis, as recurring themes within individual interview transcripts and across the collection of interviews.

A comparison of results of both sets of data demonstrated that in several instances both quantitative and qualitative findings supported the themes which emerged from the data. Within this chapter the findings are presented, theme by theme illustrating both the quantitative and qualitative datasets. The linkage of both methods is demonstrated in relation to how each dataset answered aspects of the research questions. A table defining the linkage of both data sets in the findings stage, relevant to the research questions, is included within this chapter,

The following table outlines the dominant and recurring themes and related sub themes which emerged from this study data.

5.1.1 Themes and Subthemes from both datasets

Themes	Sub Themes
Stakeholder Role	Experience
Recognition & Status	Recognition, Registration, Government oversight, Protection of therapy title. No Academic Validation No government will to engage with sector
Evidence of Effect	Scientific Evidence of effect Anecdotal clinical evidence of effect
Public Awareness and Access	Public Awareness of Regulation/Registration Public Demand and Access.
Professional Regulation	Voluntary Self - Regulation Professional Accreditation or approval of training
Employment	Job creation, Practitioners self employed Personal job satisfaction

Table 5.1: Thematic Map From Both Quantitative and Qualitative Data.

The following table outlines which sections of the study questions were addressed by either the quantitative, qualitative or both datasets, in the findings stage.

Linkage of Quantitative and Qualitative Findings

Themes	Subthemes	Quant Findings	Qual Findings
Role of CAM Stakeholders		YES	NO
	Experience	NO	YES
Recognition & Status	Recognition, Registration, Academic Validation, Government oversight, Protection of therapy title	NO	YES
Evidence of Effect	Scientific Evidence	YES	YES
	Anecdotal Evidence	YES	YES
Public Awareness and Access	Public Awareness of	YES	YES
	Regulation/Registration	NO	YES
	Public Demand and Access.		
Professional Regulation	Voluntary Self- Regulation	YES	YES
	Professional Accreditation or approval of training	YES	YES
Employment	Self -Employment	NO	YES
	Job Creation	NO	YES
	Jon Satisfaction	NO	YES

Table 5.2: Linkage of Quantitative and Qualitative Findings

Colour Code Identification Key:

Recognition & Status	Evidence of Effect	Therapy Training	Professional Regulation	Public Awareness & Demand	Employment

Table 5.3: Code identification key

The following themes which emerged from the data are discussed

5.1.2 Stakeholder Roles

This was addressed by the quantitative data collected in the questionnaire from both piloted questionnaires and the main questionnaire completed by respondents from the wider CAM community. Stakeholders who completed the questionnaire were from each section of the CAM community, as outlined in the chart below.

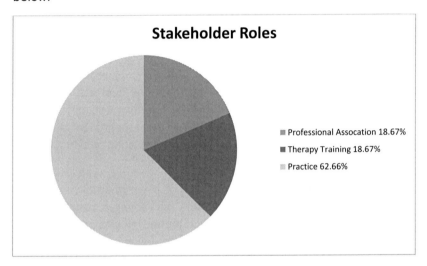

Figure 5.1: Stakeholder Roles representing educational and professional organisations

5.2 Recognition and Status

The CAM sector in Ireland has no formal or legal status, no registration of therapists, or recognition of their qualifications, and no official oversight on their training and practice. This has emerged as an issue of public safety for those who seek their training, treatments and services. This lack of recognition and professional status is replicated in the UK, EU and most of the western world.

This is supported by the data produced from both the quantitative and qualitative elements of the study and was the first dominant theme to emerge from both sets of data. It was quantified within the questionnaire responses and discussed within the interview transcripts. There are no formal regulatory structures for CAM in Ireland. Therapists are not recognised as healthcare providers and there are no national registers of therapists so members of the public seeking treatments are left very much to their own devices in sourcing therapists. There is no government oversight for the sector in terms of provision of treatment, or health and safety standards. Non-recognition of their therapy as a valid healthcare practice emerged as a strong theme throughout the responses. Recognition goes hand-in-hand with government regulatory policies and structures and the lack of government structures emerged as a dominant theme of concern for the sector. All questionnaire respondents confirmed there is no recognition of their therapy in Ireland, and no will by government agencies to engage with this sector.

Ireland is not alone in this lack of governmental structures or policies within national CAM sectors as several comments from within questionnaire text boxes confirmed a similar lack of government policy on CAM therapies, in countries other than Ireland, specifically the UK, EU and other countries of the world.

5.2.1 Recognition and Status Quantitative Findings

The following table outlines the results of Q1 the international pilot questionnaire which shows that the only countries with limited recognition for their CAM sectors are Australia and the US. No other countries have legal status or recognition for the CAM sector.

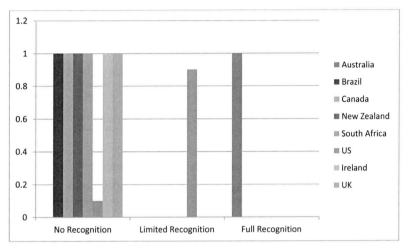

Figure 5.2: CAM Recognition Status excluding Asia and the Middle East*
* Asian countries such as China, Korea and Japan are not included in this study as there is an acceptance and integration of Eastern and Western healthcare choices within these countries.

*45 out of 50 US have limited CAM recognition; the other 5 states have no recognition.

The lack of legal status and recognition of the CAM sector in Ireland and the UK and many western countries is supported by the findings of an international review by conducted by SMCI Associates on behalf of HETAC and the DOHC on which countries had governmental structures in place for statutory regulation and therefore recognition of the CAM sector, academic validation of training programmes, the report found that only three countries in the western world had government recognition of three CAM therapies, with the accompanying legal status as healthcare professionals, academic validation of their training programmes and inclusion within the main healthcare options for the public.

135

They are:

Australia	Acupuncture/Traditional Chinese Medicine, Chiropractic, Osteopathy
New Zealand	Chiropractic, Osteopathy
UK	Chiropractic, Osteopathy

Table 5.4 SMCI (2011 Pg.. 37).

5.2.2 Recognition and Status Qualitative Findings

Qualitative data from both the questionnaire comment boxes and the stakeholder interview transcripts confirm this theme and the relation subthemes which emerged from the study. Although it could be argued that in Ireland, we have common law and under that principle, regulation need not be undertaken unless a particular need or risk is identified. The government of 2004/ 2005 National Working Group initiative on the Regulation of Complementary Therapists did identify a need for regulation for category one therapists DOHC (2005). Respondent's comments from the in-depth interviews, show that the lack of status and recognition does have a clear impact on their training and practice. Although most CAM learning providers make every effort to provide good quality training, there are reportedly a variation of training courses, where as one provider, put it *"it is difficult to see how such courses could provide safe therapists"* Interview No 9. Ireland. Lack of recognition and registration also puts restrictions on practitioner's ability to work and deliver their treatments to the public who seek out their treatments.

Some of the qualitative comments from the Q1 questionnaire comment boxes are outlined in the following table.

Brazil	"Free for all - no statutory regulation, only voluntary self-regulation"
South Africa	"In 2001, The South African government legislation of Chinese Medicine and acupuncture treatment in South Africa to legalize"
Australia	"National government recognized and Registered"*(Some therapies)
US	"In the USA, Acupuncture and Herbal Medicine is regulated at the State level and is legal in 45 of 50 States"
Canada	"Acupuncuture and Chinese Medicine is not legistated yet".
New Zealand	"There is no regulation at this moment. There is multiprofessional reccomendation from the government, but without law".

Table 5.5 Q1 Comments From Questionnaire Comment Boxes.

Respondent comments from stakeholder interviews describe recognition of their therapy and their lack of any legal status as a strong thread throughout the interviews.

Interview number four, expressed the following comment.

"We are not recognised. I cannot work in a hospital as a dietician, because I am a nutritionist not a dietician. A dietician has different training, even though the training is very similar. It does not make my qualification any less than a dieticians, just different, but no less valuable, but I can't work in a hospital . Even though I see people with diabetes. Some of my patients are children some are in the 80s, still getting the same diet sheet from the dietician, and I certainly wouldn't, I wouldn't give people the same diet sheet, as that would be a limited treatment."

A questionnaire respondent commented on the lack of recognition and a negative perception for CAM therapies

"CAM practitioners will not receive any official recognition while they are seen as "alternative" we may as well be fortune tellers" Respondent No 3.3

137

This was also discussed by a practitioner who is also involved in professional regulation of her therapy

> "Although I have met with the minister for health Dr. XX in March of this year and he did indicate that he was very interested in regulation but I think his knowledge of the whole field is quite limited. A lot of work would have to be done in raising his awareness of what goes on and the difficulties faced by practitioners in Ireland."

The lack of recognition and status was also discussed in the text boxes of the questionnaire with the following comments being typical of respondents point of view.

Comment no 5 " No legal status"

Comment No 6 "No statutory regulation of CAM therapies"

Comment No 7 "Voluntary self -regulation, no government support or registration"

5.2.3 No Government Oversight or Engagement With The Sector

This was a recurring sub theme which emerged from the data and is tied in with the broader question of recognition and status. Although successive governments have not decided on any structure or policy for the recognition of complementary therapists, the 2004 /2005 government initiative, which resulted in the publication of a report with recommendations for the regulation of Complementary Therapists, remains the only official report with recommendations for government. This report is on occasion referred to by government

138

officials although its recommendations have not been acted on. This report was referred to in interview number four with the following quotation. Since the publication of this report there has been no engagement by government agencies with the CAM sector. The fact that the professional associations are not acknowledged by government, and there is no government oversight also limits their authority and their ability to self- regulate within the sector.

Practitioners themselves discuss the need for quality oversight of their training and practice as the absence of any oversight can open to poor quality training and leave the public open to rogue practitioners, incidences of which have been documented in the media. One practitioner commented on non- recognition and non-registration of CAM training and practice.

> *"It is vital for public safety to have qualifications validated and to have practitioners registered so that they adhere to agreed code of practice and ethics"* Respondent No 3.1

The following comment was made by a CAM practitioner who also has a role as a regulator representing a population of therapists, in relation on the lack of recognition and government engagement with the sector.

> *"Well I suppose it's relevant in that it's the document that the department are aware of and until it's been replaced by something, I mean the last reprort that was done, was published in 2012 I suppose it is on pause. We don't really know if that's going anywhere".* Interview No 4 Ireland

One respondent, who had trained in Australia which does recognise some CAM therapies made the following response in terms of recognition and status.

> *"It is more difficult here, in Australia were are seen as a discrete medical profession whereas here we are seen as alternative, not even complimentary so it seems to me here you have doctors, physiotherapists, who work in mainstream medicine and there are a few doctors who have referred to me medically, but I wouldn't say that osteopathy is considered part of the main healthcare community or medical community"* Interview No 10 Ireland.

In comparing the CAM status between Ireland and the UK, there was also the lack of government policy and structure for the regulation of CAM therapies in the UK. One of the UK respondents made the following comment

> *"There is no statutory status in the UK yet although heated discussion for this has been going over 12 years"* Interview No 14 UK.

This is also confirmed by the respondent from Spain, who had the following comment.

> *"CAM Medicine are not regulated in Spain and from Ministry of Health is interpreted that only western doctors can practise it. However, there is a huge tolerance as it demonstrate the matter that 1.200 of the approximated 15.000 professionals who practise it, are western doctors. Nowadays, it does exists a health commission which is making a study (demanded from*

the Spanish Parliament) about this matter as a possible way for a future regulation" Interview No.19 Spain.

The following comment from an interview from a learning provider and practitioner confirmed that there is no regulation for CAM therapies in Brazil.

"Everyone can practise in Brazil as there is no regulation. It is in our constitution that you cannot force someone to do or not do something if there is no law" Interview No 20 Brazil.

5.2.4 No Protection of Therapy Title

There is no protection of title for qualified CAM therapists in any discipline and any individual, regardless of background or training can describe themselves as a CAM therapist without sanction. This is one of the sub themes, linked to recognition and status of CAM therapies which emerged from the interview transcripts. Protection of title had not been included as a question within the questionnaire but had emerged from interview transcripts as a strong sub theme to the broader theme on recognition and status. The Irish professional associations have long been seeking protection of title for their therapies. This is particularly relevant when therapies have agreed their training standards and they wish to protect those standards. Within the current regulation vacuum, there is nothing to stop any individual practising any therapy of which they may have little or in some cases, no formal training in and describe themselves as a professional therapist. Voluntary professional bodies can only regulate their own members and they currently have no sanction over this practice. Some of the interviewees described incidences when healthcare therapists who would do short training courses in a particular therapy, sometimes of less than 10% of what the well trained therapist would have done, and then practice that therapy in whatever limited way, using that therapy title. That has been reported by acupuncture bodies who complain that other therapists can do the one weekend's training in needling skills, or auricular therapy and then describe themselves as acupuncturists, offer an Acupuncture service as an adjunctive to a healthcare treatment. It is also reported by other therapies such as osteopaths and chiropractors that healthcare professionals can do short training courses in a therapy and then describe themselves as osteopaths or chiropractors. Some of the interview participants referred to this in the following comments.

"It's very frustrating to see one weekend courses for health professionals being advertised as dry needling and then to see these offering acupuncture treatments to their patients on the basis of one weekend training. It's a real issue of public safety and is damaging to us as a profession who have agreed our basic training standards within the profession" Interview No 9 Ireland.

This is also replicated by another interview respondent who made the following comment.

"I think it comes down to our practice and protection of title for of our profession. I think what you see in Europe is that osteopathy has become polarised. So the people who are X and Y are also adopting an adjunctive education in osteopathy and working as osteopaths, or using a number of different expressions or descriptions. I doubt if this serves the profession of osteopathy" Interview No 10 Ireland.

Learning Providers, regulators and practitioners interviewed on this topic as the comments demonstrate expressed a frustration on the lack of a single agreed standard for their therapy and the lack of the ability to enforce breaches of standards. There are no figures to hand with regard to of health professionals who undertake short CAM courses as adjunctive training as, as this areas has yet to be studied, and the comments are from stakeholders own experiences.

5.3 Evidence of Effect

There is a body of scientific research for some CAM therapies, although many therapies rely on informal anecdotal clinical evidence from their practitioners to demonstrate evidence of effect.

A dominant and recurring theme to emerge from both qualitative and qualitative data is the role of evidence of effective treatment in practice and in presenting the case for regulation. This was also cited in the 2012, SMCI report which had been commissioned by a joint committee of members of both the DOHC, and HETAC, as a requirement for consideration of the establishment of a regulation framework for this sector. There is a diversity of therapies, and although several of the primary therapies have justified their treatments through a body of scientific and clinical evidence there is a perception of CAM therapies which links all therapies together including the weaker less proven therapies, which in turn presents difficulties for the sector in terms of cohesion.

Although the complexity of the range of CAM therapies has been addressed within the National Working Group Report on the Regulation of Complementary Therapists in terms of categorising therapies, the perception remains and has been cited by government as a consideration in deciding on a framework for regulation. The following chart outlines questionnaire results on evidence of effect of their therapy.

5.3.1 Evidence of Effect Quantitative Findings

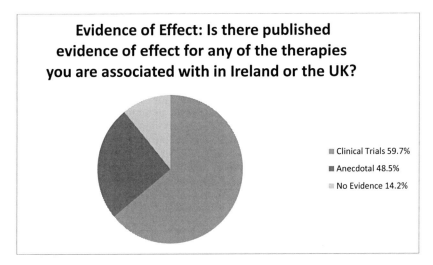

Evidence of Effect: Is there published evidence of effect for any of the therapies you are associated with in Ireland or the UK?

- Clinical Trials 59.7%
- Anecdotal 48.5%
- No Evidence 14.2%

Figure 5.3: Evidence of Effect Q3 Findings

*Please note that some respondents chose more than one option as in some cases there are both clinical and anecdotal evidence of effect.

Questionnaire data demonstrated that the CAM sector is aware of the significance of evidence of effect of their treatments, and respondents were aware of whether there was scientific evidence, anecdotal evidence gathered from clinical reports or both.

5.3.2 Evidence of Effect Qualitative Findings

Interview transcripts supported quantitative findings and demonstrated evidence of effect of their treatments, whether through scientific trials or clinical evidential reports and records. Several of the respondents interviewed discussed patient satisfaction and treatment benefit within their interviews. These are some of the comments from respondent interviews, when asked about research and evidence of effect for their therapy.

"Yes there is a body of research. We have put a link on our website is in this to numerous controlled trials, which are linked to our website" Interview number 10 Ireland.

One of the long-standing learning providers in Ireland when asked about evidence of effect spoke about how rewarding it was to see graduates of her training programme publishing evidence of good treatment effect on the websites. She made the following comment.

"It's very rewarding when you see graduates working in busy practices and you see patients putting confirmatory comments on their websites and complimenting them on good effect after successful treatments" Interview No 3 Ireland.

CAM treatments are surviving and in some countries growing because of evidence of good effect. In a recent two centre, London and Dublin, study in which patients were asked why they continued to seek CAM treatments, especially in London, where healthcare treatments are free on the NHS, they indicated that they come because they find the treatments effective, Ward (2009).

Another interviewee, who is a learning provider and provides clinical treatments, confirmed that there is good evidence of effect of treatment, and this is demonstrated by the growth in patients seeking and paying for CAM treatments, when public health care is free in Brazil. He made the following comments

"More and more, there was a study that said there was a growth of about 400%In Brazil the public health system is always free, so they keep track of everything that they do. So they compared how many people got acupuncture five years ago and last year" Interview number 20 Brazil.

Comments on evidence of effect of treatments were also included within the questionnaire by respondents who added their own comments within the text boxes provided.

These are comments from respondents 3 and 4 on evidence of effect for their therapies.

"Evidence of efficacy of individual herbs and other natural remedies e.g. on PubMed etc"(Respondent 3).

"Herbal Medicine has many trials published" Respondent 4.

Several other respondents also commented on evidence of effect for their therapies. This was one of the comment boxes within the questionnaire which many respondents completed. The following comments are a sample of their responses regarding evidence of effect of their therapies.

"Lots of evidence on healthy nutrition and save the day, and efficacy of herbal medicines available, usually through organisational websites" Respondent 5.

"There are many published trials for acupuncture has been the subject of research" Respondent 6.

"Some research on craniosacral therapy also" Respondent 7.

"RCTs cannot be used for herbs as used by herbalists, herbs have multiple active constituents. RCTs need to be refined before they can be used on herbs. Herbs have been around

147

for a long time, caveat emptor; people wouldn't use them if they didn't work" Respondent 20.

"RFI Reiki Federation Ireland has anecdotal evidence" Respondent 11.

"it was agreed by M. H. Minister for health that anecdotal evidence is considered as evidence, this was due mainly to the high volume of anecdotal evidence available for Reiki and the government is unable to fund controlled trials" Respondent 24.

5.4. CAM Therapy Training

CAM therapy training is primarily delivered by private providers in Ireland, feeding the market for CAM therapists. The majority of training courses have no external quality oversight of their training content and delivery. This is a common model of CAM training in many western countries.

Survey results showed that 87.5% of complementary therapies are offered by private individuals or groups, representing a variety of CAM students and graduates. Discussion on therapy training, academic validation in Ireland and outside of Ireland was a strong theme running throughout the interviews and the questionnaire comment text boxes. The absence of formal regulatory structures impacted on therapy training in that currently there is no academic validation or recognition of any CAM therapy in Ireland, and therefore no formal Irish quality oversight of program content or delivery. 35.5% of respondents surveyed reported that they sought external validation of their training courses outside of Ireland. Quality oversight of their training programs was facilitated by the external validators.

5.4.1 Academic Quantitative Findings

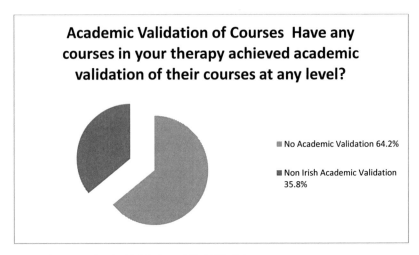

Academic Validation of Courses Have any courses in your therapy achieved academic validation of their courses at any level?

■ No Academic Validation 64.2%

■ Non Irish Academic Validation 35.8%

Figure 5.4: Academic Validation of CAM Training

5.4.2 Academic Validation Qualitative Findings

The lack of academic validation and therefore recognition of their training courses were strong themes throughout the qualitative data on this subject, and confirm the quantitative findings. CAM learning providers share many attributes in that the majority of them have learned one or more, complimentary therapies. Data recorded from interviews shows that there is a high degree of motivation, and a high degree of investment in terms of time, effort and personal funds from many of the learning providers. Many of them would not have had teacher training previously, and would have in fact "learned on the job" however, several of them spoke of the personal time commitment and responsibility they have undertaken in order to deliver their training programmes. Data from interview transcripts shows that they sought guidance from anywhere it was available, both inside and outside of Ireland. One interviewee who has become

150

a successful Learning Provider spoke about the early setup of her course, and made the following comments.

"No, which is terrible to say really, it's terrible to admit. I didn't do any specific course. I had a mentor I suppose, I kind of didn't think there was anything available you know...... I feel certainly that the mentor I had, who was from FAS, she would have a had a Masters in training at that stage and she was a client of mine, we got on really well and she would have helped me in the design of the course, in writing learning outcomes, so like 20 years ago, we had it broken up into Modules, which is what they do now, and we were writing learning outcomes at that stage. So that was a good start and I'm not sure if our assessments were properly in line with our learning outcomes because that's probably relevant" Interview 1 Ireland.

They created employment, employing experts, as reported in the early stages of set up of their courses from either the UK or other countries where training programs in their therapy would already have been established. The following comment describes how Learning Providers sought experts in their area to help prepare and deliver their courses

"We would have looked for the top people we could find in those areas. So for a number of years I felt that area was looked after so that my area was supporting teachers and becoming more involved in the practical aspect of it and in the clinics" Interview 1 Ireland.

In many cases they sought academic validation of their qualifications, guidance on accreditation and engaged with the Department of education and the various government agencies responsible for higher education, over long periods of time. The following comment represents a typical example of the experience of one such Learning Provider who spoke about the early days in starting her course.

"Well, I guess when I started the course to be brutally honest, I had no idea what I was taking on. And I think that if it had not

151

been for my partner, who has put a lot into the course and has been a lot of support I would not have been able to continue. I think that the course provides two full-time jobs with lots of unpaid overtime. We have not made any money. Everything we have made on the course we have put right back into the course and the college and our accountant can attest to that. We have had to invest a huge amount of money into putting the academic material online and to paying experts to deliver some of the material online and to pay experts to deliver the material and the technology we've invested huge amounts into the technology and my partner works 24 seven on this. I think it's taken everything. It's been everything. It's not just a vocation, but it is takes everything" Interview No 3 Ireland

Lack of course validation and any official quality oversight cannot fail to have an impact on the quality and consistency of courses in various CAM therapies being delivered, and this cannot fail to have an impact on the quality and consistency of therapists in the marketplace offering healthcare treatments to the public. Individual providers discuss their own standards which they implement themselves in their own training programs. These are some of the comments from questionnaire text boxes. The following comment does not refer to academic validation of training, but to a membership standard of a professional association, as in line with many other therapies, a professional membership standard is the only quality oversight available in Ireland.

"In shiatsu practitioners are accredited individually having first satisfied a set of criteria of attendance as a course of sufficient duration with specified curricula. Respondent 3

The following comment refers to external validation and accreditation of therapy training through a non-Irish organisation.

"Rigorous process of training to certification and overseen by the American Holistic Nurses Association for Credentialing. This therapy was started by nurses in Denver, Colorado in the 80s" Respondent 4.

Interview respondents spoke of training outside of Ireland when no training in that particular therapy was available in Ireland. This respondent refers to training in Scotland, which together with England and other parts of the UK has academic validation and recognition of CAM training programs and qualifications.

"There was my course, at the Scottish school, and then I applied and I did a preliminary year from 1998 to 1999, and then I started the degree program properly in 99 to 2000, and that year they had gotten validation. So in between starting just doing an introductory thing to the sciences as a refresher and actually going on to the degree they validated it so I emerged, I enrolled in a degree program and emerged with a degree" Respondent No 2.

Some Irish CAM learning providers interviewed spoke about applying for HETAC validation of their programs, when it was available in Ireland to CAM providers between 2005 and 2008. They discussed the process of going through the application and their efforts and work, to meet higher education standard. They spoke about their difficulties. When this process was halted by HETAC and how these impacted on their training programs and students.

"There is no government accreditation by the Department of education or validation and I was very heavily involved in preparation for course validation with HETAC. We met all the requirements but then at the very last minute, the Council decided not to validate because it might be cutting across the Department of Health as far as I'm aware. We are the only

academic programme in Ireland ever to be stopped, having met all the requirements" Interview No 9 Ireland.

"I lecture with X, we spent months and lots of hard work to bring our course to degree level, we were approved but unfortunately have still not been granted the degree status" Respondent No 26

When asked about quality standards of CAM training respondents made the following comments

"The fact that there are no quality standards for this sector and we are stuck in limbo because there has been no activity and people who don't suffer are the people who have a lesser quality course, because there's no agreed academic standard between associations. No oversight, and it's an issue of public safety as people go to courses that do not have training standards and you know it's difficult to see how they can produce good practitioners, public safety is an issue" Interview No 9 Ireland.

"I would like to see better standards of education generally. As a therapist and employer, I have seen dramatic variances in student standards who have the same qualifications but from different colleges" Respondent No 18.

Another Irish CAM learning provider made the following comment on his attempts to apply for validation of his course in homoeopathy.

"We did approach HETAC here regarding validation of our course but there were obstacles to having a course in Homeopathy validated. There have been problems in a number of other countries also regarding validation. Successful graduates have the option of taking a Master's

programme MSc, in the University of Central Lancashire if they wish" Interview No 7 Ireland.

Another learning provider discussed their experience with regard to academic validation of their training programme.

"Academically, right now, there is no accrediting body by any accrediting body I mean, HETAC or QQI They don't recognise complimentary medicine if they do decide to in the future, I think I would look at the possibility of going through that process again. Probably this time, I would like to do it independently, so we would become independently validated rather than attached to another institution. I'm not sure, I would have to look at the situation, but at the moment there is no process, there is nothing we can do here in Ireland to academically validate unless we look at linking or looking for validation with an English university or the University of Wales. I don't think it's necessary. I'm happy with the course that it's a high standard" interview No 3 Ireland

The following respondents spoke about the importance of having some process of recognition and validation for a CAM training course, so that their certification would give them confidence in practice.

"Without a valid course, we are just wasting our time doing the course without the validation and accreditation. I would not be confident in selling myself to a client or potential business partner" Respondent No 21.

"Training is expensive and money and time there has to be some validation to ensure the quality and their knowledge is sufficient for the work" Respondent number 10.

155

Learning Providers who completed comment boxes within the questionnaire commented on the impact that a lack of validation of training programmes has on their sector, their students and graduates.

> *"By removing the academic award standards for CAM Training or training courses and Ireland are now liable for VAT and that which is making it uncompetitive to train here. We don't have the option of being recognised" Respondent No 23.*

> *"All education and training, regardless of subject should have a route to academic validation, I believe an academic standard of education should be shown to get validated" Respondent number 24.*

Those comments directly represent the opinions of both the successful and smaller Learning Providers and the therapists who seek training.

5.5 Public Access and Awareness

The issue of public demand for CAM therapies has been addressed in the literature review and was not a question within the questionnaire. It was however one of the guide questions within the interviews and several interviewees commented on the demand for their treatments and services. Public awareness of the recognition, regulation and registration of CAM therapies, was included in the questionnaire, and produced the following results.

5.5.1 Public Access and Awareness Quantitative Findings

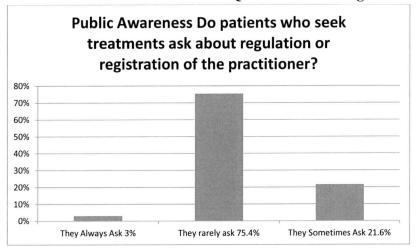

Figure 5.5: Public Awareness Quantitative Findings.

These results demonstrate that public "rarely ask" about regulation or registration of therapists they seek treatments from. Qualitative data from stakeholder interviews and comment boxes provide broader data on this topic.

5.5.2 Public Access and Awareness Qualitative Findings

Respondents also reported that members of the public consistently seek CAM treatments and the lack of a professional register means that they will try to find one themselves. There is no official register to consult, and no information on training or qualifications to help them make a judgement on choice of therapist or treatment. Practitioners interviewed for this study report that their patients very often ask among their own family and friends for a recommendation to a particular therapist, without any checking of expertise, qualifications or safety. This viewpoint was replicated in several of the interviews as, reportedly there is a consistent public demand for treatments and patients are obliged to do their own research if they cannot get a recommendation from somebody they know, in many cases by just asking around. Interview number 3 made the following comment, that patients want a treatment and will try to seek a recommendation from anybody they can. They attend the therapist with the assumption that the therapist is properly trained and is a safe therapist, which is mostly the case, as most registered therapists are competent, responsible and safe, however the lack of oversight leaves this open to abuse, both in terms of healthcare and patient finance.

"In my experience, people in Ireland have a very innate understanding of natural healing of any of kind, and they tend to go to a therapist or practitioner of any kind based on recommendations of their friends, family and their broader circle.. Basically, it's word-of-mouth. I have never had to advertise and it's probably best practice not to advertise, but we have always found our patients or clients by word-of-mouth personal recommendations, so they come to you, having been told by so-and-so that go to whatever name. She is very good for arthritis and they don't look for certificates, I have my certificate, of course, and I have never bothered to hang it. I have rarely been questioned by anybody. I think they presume when they come to your clinic that you are well trained and well experienced" Interview No 3.Ireland.

One interview participant who has a history of involvement in professional regulation as well as being an experienced practitioner when asked if patients question her qualifications or registration made the following reply

"Not at all, they don't honestly give a hoot. I mean I have my qualifications up on the wall and every now and then someone might distractedly look at them while I'm sort of, you know, doing something else but really they just want to know it's going to work" Interview no 2, Ireland.

Some CAM treatments are invasive, such as acupuncture, and manipulative, such as chiropractic and osteopathy, and are not without risk, as had been indicated in the National Working Group Report on the Regulation of Complementary Therapists DOHC(2005). Another interview respondent made the following comment when asked about whether patients question registration qualifications.

"I think most of our patients come from word-of-mouth. Usually they would know somebody who we have helped and they come would come under that basis" Interview number 10 Ireland

5.5.3 Public Access to CAM Therapies

CAM therapies are paid for by patients seeking treatment and there is no policy of public access to treatments in Ireland. Only those patients who can afford treatments have access to a range of treatments as the CAM sector operates within the private healthcare sector, both in terms of training and practice. This was one of the sub themes which emerged from the dominant theme of Public Awareness and was discussed by some of the respondents as being important to the benefit of the patient and to their own livelihood. In reality, there is no publicly financed access to CAM therapies. All patients pay for treatments which are typically carried out in private clinics, sometimes at the therapists own home or in professional rooms or shared multidisciplinary clinics. The lack of government oversight for a diversity of therapies delivering treatments to the public is an issue of concern and of public safety. Many of the respondents commented on this issue within questionnaire text boxes and within the interview transcripts. While the voluntary professional bodies have some sort of oversight of their members, the lack of any regulatory responsibility does create a safety gap.

"There should be resident acupuncturists in every hospital as it is very good for pain relief and lots of things that can't be dealt with"

"I think there should be more emphasis on preventative medicine and I think even in these recessionary times, it would save money if the government invested in prevention of disease. We should be in all of these centres. These new centres of excellence that Mr X keeps talking about, and we should be at the coalface of healthcare" Interview No 4 Ireland.

Although there is no public access to complementary therapies in public facilities in Ireland, there is limited access in the National

Health Service in the UK. The lack of public access to complementary therapies is no barrier to members of the public seeking and paying for treatments in Ireland. Those who can afford to, seek out and pay for treatments. Writing in a paper for the Irish College of General Practitioners, Dr. Michael Maguire outlined the following statistics on use of Therapies in Europe.

"The use of complementary medicine is growing rapidly in Europe. 50% of French and Germans use some type of it. In France, homoeopathy is used by 36% of patients (from 16% in 1982). In Denmark, reflexology is the most popular alternative modality. In Belgium, France and the Netherlands it's homoeopathy, while in Sweden, the UK and the USA osteopathic and chiropractic therapies are at the forefront. Acupuncture is also very popular in most European countries. In Germany, 77% of pain clinics use acupuncture. In Belgium, conventional medical practitioners carry out 84% of the homoeopathy and 74% of acupuncture treatments. In the Netherlands, 47% of medical doctors use some form of complementary medicine, Maguire (2004 Pg. 3).

In Ireland those who have private health insurance can claim some rebates from the health insurers if they receive treatments from a therapists who is a member of a professional association which has been approved by the health insurers. (VHI website) This has been discussed in an earlier chapter, and is referred to by Maguire (ICGP).

"if a GP or consultant refers a patient to a complementary practitioner then the fees are allowable. VHI and BUPA allow the same concessions" Ibid.

In the UK, as discussed, there is some acceptance of CAM therapies within NHS hospitals, although this seems to have been initiated on an individual hospital basis, rather than as an overall policy of inclusion. Interview respondents indicate that the hospital authorities are supportive, and limited CAM therapies will be included for as long as hospital support continues. It seems to be discretionary, according to indications from interview respondents.

The following extract from a UK interview confirms this.

> *S. I was using it (acupuncture) in Plymouth hospital maternity hospital, this was 1988*
>
> *B. Was this totally acceptable, did you need to get permissions?*
>
> *S. Yes I had consultants who were supportive and saw it was effective, so said "give it a go". The head of midwifery was also very supportive and very excited that we were doing something innovative, so that was good",* Interview No 16 UK.

This interviewee reported that when a change of hospital management occurred, this practice was discontinued and acupuncture, which had been available at this unit for fifteen years and was found by patients to be effective, is no longer offered as part of this unit

5.6 Professional Regulation

Voluntary Professional Associations are the only route to access public information on CAM therapies and the only therapy representation in Ireland. This is also the case in the UK, EU and most western countries.

Data received from both quantitative and qualitative elements of this study have demonstrated that voluntary self-regulating professional bodies provide the only public access to information on CAM Therapies, and are the only representative structures for CAM Therapies in Ireland.

Quantitative findings are outlined in chart format in the following page.

5.6.1 Professional Regulation Quantitative Findings

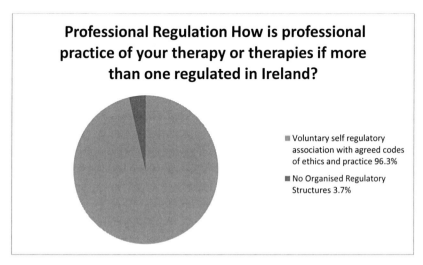

Figure 5.6: Professional Regulation in Ireland

Voluntary self- regulatory structures have been set up in Ireland and in other countries, primarily by the therapists themselves, sometimes by the learning providers and in several cases by a combination of both. The typical model of the professional association, is a voluntary self-regulatory body which is operated and governed by member therapists. While some of the professional bodies have incorporated, many of them have registered names and function with the companies' office without formally incorporating. Most of the professional associations today have public information websites which publishes their standards of membership and practice. Professional associations typically have an agreed constitution, which guides their functionality. They have agreed codes of ethics

163

and practice to guide their therapist members, in many cases, offer public information and in most cases handle complaints from the public. All of these standards within their codes of ethics and practice are self- imposed and self –regulated. At the moment they have no function of regulation or representation for their therapy outside of their membership, and there is no route of complaint for rogue therapists other than to advise a complainant to refer to the police in the event of a serious complaint against a therapist who is not a member of the association. A limited number of CAM therapies negotiated treatment rebates with the private health insurance companies in the mid-nineties, for their registered members, which is a benefit to those offering treatments and to the patients who are members of those health insurance schemes. This remains the only inspection and approval system for any CAM therapy in Ireland.

Many associations, as stated earlier, are long established and have been representing their members with various government agencies for several years. They have received no guidance or facilitation or in some cases even acknowledgement by government of their activities on behalf of the therapies and are fully funded by membership subscriptions. There officers and board members elected at AGM typically are working therapists and are not paid for their regulatory work, but can in some cases seek payment for expenses in carrying out their duties. In many CAM disciplines, there are more than one Professional Association, representing therapists of the same discipline. There is no official criteria for the establishment of a professional association and if a group of therapists do not like the format and structure of an association in their own discipline, they can choose to establish another association. Therefore there can be several associations in one CAM discipline with no agreed educational or practice standards between the associations.

5.6.2 Professional Regulation Qualitative Findings

The role of the professional association was also a dominant theme within the qualitative interviews, and some respondents discussed their standards and functions and their oversight on training and practice in Ireland, as an example of a global model. Some respondent indications are that in some disciplines there is broad agreement on standards between different associations, although it is also reported that this is not always the case.

"Each discipline has its own association with no link between standards as therapies differ" Respondent 12.

"In herbal medicine there are particular traditions such as Western, Chinese and Ayurvedic and respective associations have formed for each. This does not mean that herbal medicine is fractured but that different PAs represent different traditions" Respondent 17.

"There are two professional associations involved" Respondent 10.

The following comment in from a practitioner who also has a voluntary role in a professional association, representing a body of professional therapists. When asked about the role of the association. She made the following comment.

"It regulates, and is responsible for the regulation of a register of acupuncturists it is the oldest Association of its kind in Ireland. It regulates practice, gives information to its members. It gives information to the public. It provides insurance for its members and deals with any queries from the

public. It organises continuing professional development for its members and provides guidelines and information on that. There is also a requirement that members hold first aid qualifications. It monitors these certificates for members. We are very professional and our standards are very high"
Interview No 4 Ireland

As previously stated, and is demonstrated by the questionnaire responses the majority of CAM disciplines have their professional associations, or more than one in some instances. Learning providers and training programs are all major stakeholders within the whole CAM community, as without the provision of graduates, the associations could not continue and without some form of registration of their graduates, the learning providers would have similar difficulties. It could be argued that professional associations and private learning providers of all CAM therapies are mutually dependent. The following interview respondent who is a learning provider, when asked about the Professional Association or her therapy made the following comment.

"Yes, we have an association called the Irish Association of Master Medical Herbalists, which is made up of graduates, not only of our course, but of other courses in the tradition. Some members would have trained years ago in England and they live and work here, so they are members of our association. That association has been around for more than 14 years. It was set up before we started our school I was a member of the board as a younger person, and it recently became affiliated to the XY a group of organisations in England who represent herbal associations of different traditions within the EU" Interview No 3.Ireland

In the UK and other countries with strong CAM communities, professional associations in the various disciplines are also prevalent. The results of the UK questionnaire had several commonalities with the previous questionnaires sent to CAM stakeholders in Ireland internationally and the EU. The UK, as previously discussed, does have academic validation and that is twinned with academic recognition of the training programmes, so learners receive a recognised qualification on completion of their training. There is, however, still no recognition of any CAM therapy in the UK as a healthcare practice. There is no government policy on recognition, regulation or registration of therapists. The professional associations have been very active in the different disciplines of engaging with government. The UK government have engaged directly with professional associations in therapies identified as being necessary to have a regulation structure. They are however moving away from statutory regulation, towards self-regulation for some of these disciplines. One of the UK interview respondents made the following comments when discussing the current status of the lack of regulation in the UK.

"The current focus is herbal because the government has already decided against regulating, acupuncture, and they have already shifted their attention away and they encouraged the X Y Council to join the professional standards agency and they are voluntarily regulated. So they have already passed their assessment and have been granted to join the professional standards agency" Interview No 14 UK.

The respondents from Holland and Spain also discussed the lack of government oversight of CAM therapies in Holland and Spain. The only quality oversight in Holland is carried out by Private Health Insurance Companies, who have set a practice standard, responding to public demand of inclusion of CAM therapies within their health insurance policies.

The respondent from Holland made the following comment.

"There's no official status, so everybody can practice whatever they want, irrespective of their level of training. So the difference is if you are trained properly, if you are a member of associations that meet the standard set by the insurance companies, not by the government, so if the association meets the criteria from the insurance company, a member of that association, the cost of their service is reimbursed, to a certain degree not 100 percent of it" Interview No 18 Holland.

When asked about the role and function of professional associations in his country, the respondent from Brazil indicated there were many professional associations, and there was no criteria for deciding what qualities that professional association should have. The Brazilian respondent is a learning provider and indicated that he is also involved within his own professional association. He made the following comment

"There are many yes, because in Brazil to open an association it's very easy. There is no official accreditation, everyone can start one. What we have is a Union of practitioners in my state, which I am on the board of" Interview No 20. Brazil.

5.6.3 Professional Accreditation of CAM Training Courses

Professional associations do provide some quality oversight of practitioner training as part of their membership standards and membership requirements. This was also a dominant sub theme from both data sets, the quantitative element of the questionnaire and the qualitative interviews and comment text boxes. Data received from closed questions within the questionnaire indicated that most respondents confirmed that there was professional self-regulation for their therapy and some process of professional accreditation for their courses, and this is presented in a quantitative findings chart on the following page.

168

5.6.4 Professional Accreditation Quantitative Findings

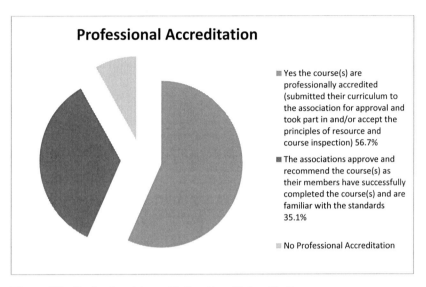

Professional Accreditation

- Yes the course(s) are professionally accredited (submitted their curriculum to the association for approval and took part in and/or accept the principles of resource and course inspection) 56.7%

- The associations approve and recommend the course(s) as their members have successfully completed the course(s) and are familiar with the standards 35.1%

- No Professional Accreditation

Figure 5.7: Professional Accreditation Quantitative Findings.

According to the responses the professional associations provide some measure of accreditation for their training programs. This varies from discipline to discipline as some CAM therapies have well organised structures and a separate course accreditation process, while others set standards of training duration and curricula and approve the graduates from courses that meet those standards for membership of their professional association.

Whatever method is used for professional accreditation or approval of CAM training, it is the only process available to CAM learning providers and students of these programs in Ireland. As such, much of the comments from both questionnaire and interview respondents indicate that professional oversight is a welcome process for all of the CAM stakeholders.

169

5.6.5 Professional Accreditation Qualitative Findings

When asked about professional quality oversight and professional regulation or approval of training programs, one interview respondent involved with regulation made the following response.

> *"Yes, we are first in bringing out the Irish X accreditation board and the colleges are required to meet our standards in order to get professional accreditation of their courses and meet our standards. We get independent inspectors to inspect the colleges to make sure that the colleges meet the standards in order to maintain their accreditation in that way we make sure that the colleges meet the standards and we are able to recommend that students go to an accredited college"* Interview No 4 Ireland.

When asked about professional accreditation or oversight of their program, the respondent from Brazil said that this was not necessary, it was not a requirement. He also made the following comments regarding internal quality in terms of health and safety, rather than training standards.

> *"Normally we do that informally because there is no necessity. We try to do that in terms of protective measures for the students, biohazard etc"* Interview No. 20 Brazil.

5.7 Employment in the CAM Sector

The CAM community creates a significant employment sector in Ireland, the UK, the EU and in countries across the world who train and practice CAM therapies. The sector provides employment for its practitioners, teachers, learning providers and regulators.

One of the emergent themes from all qualitative data from this study was that complementary therapies are a significant area of private employment. Graduates from a diversity of courses establish themselves as therapists within the private healthcare sector. They establish themselves as sole traders, or in some cases more formal structures, such as companies. Set up costs are reportedly in many cases, self- funding, either using their own funds or through personal loans or bank loans which they use to open their clinics or centres and they effectively become small businesses operators. This then feeds into the rental, supply and financial sectors, as graduates of CAM courses, establish their clinics, across countries who have such communities.

5.7.1 Employment Qualitative Data

Some practitioners report that they approach the opening of their clinic in the same way any business operation begins, and as reported by some of the respondents, adopt or source business skills to help them manage their clinic marketing, finance and business operation. This is a comment from a recently graduated practitioner.

"I was always interested in human therapies for myself.... I found I liked reflexology, so I studied it is. I also wanted to be self-employed. I researched the college and liked it" Interview No 12 Ireland.

When asked if she was making a living from her practice, she made the following comment

"Yes I think so, I am very optimistic. I just cover myself the moment I have just started, its my fifth month and I've never been in business before. So for me to be doing this, it pushes me to go forward, I have signed up to a business setup course to help me run the practice" Interview No 12 Ireland.

Job satisfaction has been a significant secondary theme running throughout the interview data. The satisfaction of being able to have the skills to deliver a therapeutic treatment and help someone with a condition they are having difficulty with, gives, as reported immense job satisfaction, When asked why she studied a CAM therapy and why is she now working in her practice, and what benefits she got from her work other than financial, she made the following response.

> *"Yes huge, huge benefits, personal satisfaction, when you get a good treatment response it makes it all worthwhile" Interview No 12, Ireland.*

This sentiment has been replicated by several of the respondents both in the interviews and the questionnaire text boxes. The aspect of working autonomously, independently and the job satisfaction they achieved when there was good patient feedback and good evidence of effect of the treatments they delivered.

> *"Yes, you do get benefits personal satisfaction from helping people and seeing people getting good effect from your treatments and seeing how the natural order of things work .I enjoy that side of things, the philosophy of osteopathy, that's my life ethos and how it works" Interview No 12 Ireland.*

The following response is from one of the Irish Learning Providers when discussing the job satisfaction she gets from delivering her course and training practitioners.

> *"With time, we probably will make a reasonable living and it's been very rewarding for me personally, but has been very exhausting" Interview No 3, Ireland.*

One of the questions asked in stakeholder interviews was concerning their future plans for investment in their future within the

172

CAM sector and in response to this question, one respondent made the following comment.

> "Yes, we're just there taken on a new receptionist are taking on another room. Another osteopath will work with us. So yes, we are investing in the future. Certainly it's an ongoing concern and we will continue to invest in it. I can't see us engaging in any other field of practice" Interview No 10 Ireland.

The common element derived from both data sets is that learning providers and practitioners have a strong motivation towards self-employment and towards working independently. One well-established practitioner, who became a learning provider made the following comments.

> "I guess my strong desire though was to have a job that had a lot of satisfaction...
>
> So there was probably 6 years really from when I qualified as a Medical Massage Therapist to when I actually started as an Osteopath. Then we set the school up in January of 1990 which was the beginning of when I was studying Osteopathy. And the big reason for the school was, I suppose it was because I was trying to find something that, I knew I needed to be learning an awful lot more and I was aware that articulating that I needed to be engaged in life- long learning and having attended a college in America where there would be post grad stuff, there was nothing here. But a huge thing was I felt I don't want to have to be going abroad all the time training so I want something centered here, whereby experts come here to me" Interview No 1 Ireland.

This experience was typical of learning providers, who invited experts in particular therapies to come to Ireland and lecture students and bring their expertise with them and many of the learning providers confirmed this to be the case. When asked about

173

creating employment the following learning provider made the following comment on employing lecturers on his course.

*"We were providing a course in Chinese medicine, and it made sense that our lecturers were experts in Chinese medicine, who came to Ireland to offer their expertise, which was not available here. We invested quite a lot of student's fees into buying this expertise, while at the same time, employing local teachers. so yes we did create employment "*Interview No 9 Ireland.

Data from all sections of this community, Learning Providers, Regulators and Practitioners have demonstrated that this sector provides employment for all stakeholders, and has the potential to create further employment should the sector receive some support and recognition from government agencies, in Ireland and elsewhere. Both datasets produced supporting data to answer the research questions.

Both Quantitative and Qualitative data, as stated answered aspects of the research questions, as defined in the following table.

Role and Experience	Quantitative Data	
No Recognition & Regulation		Qualitative Data
Quality Oversight Training and Practice	Quantitative Data	Qualitative Data
External Validation	Quantitative Data	Qualitative Data
Issues, Concerns and Needs	Quantitative Data	Quantitative Data

Table 5.14: Study Questions addressed by both quantitative and qualitative data.

Chapter 6 Discussion and Recommendations

6.1 Introduction

This study began as an investigation into the CAM community in Ireland and evolved into needs analysis for this sector. It quickly became evident that the CAM Ireland model in terms of training and practice, was typical of many countries globally. It explored many aspects of this community, including its historical background and its relationship within the Adult and Higher education sector in Ireland. Second chance education and life-long learning is a feature of CAM training, and many CAM graduates have demonstrated that the skills they acquire within the diversity of their training programmes make them employable either in the self- employed sector or the wider job marketplace. The study explored the demand for and the practice of CAM therapies and focused on the experiences of those who practice, those who teach and those who regulate this community. The historical context of this community is relevant to this study as it puts into context, the roots and the organisational beginnings of what has now become a vibrant CAM community in Ireland. Using a mixed methods research strategy of questionnaire, text box comments and in-depth interviews, the study produced a body of information which informed the research and helped to answer the research questions. As the stakeholders who contributed to this study have representative roles in the CAM sector, across a variety of therapies, a population of CAM students, graduates and practitioners have been represented in this study.

Some of the data derived from the study was expected, and as previously mentioned confirmatory, in that it is common knowledge within the CAM community that there are no regulatory policies in Ireland for this sector. Additionally, it is also common knowledge that most complementary therapy training in Ireland is provided by private providers. What was not known was the impact of the lack of

175

recognition and regulation on all sections of this community, in terms of the provision of training and practice. The failure of adult learners to get acknowledgement and recognition for their training is unique to the CAM sector and is an area which needs to be addressed by the relevant government agencies. The challenges which meet the voluntary professional groups in the self-regulation of CAM disciplines, without government support, guidance or national authority is a concern for public safety as there is no national oversight of training or practice for any CAM discipline.

Unexpected themes emerged from the study as teachers and practitioners spoke about a different philosophy of life, whether that refers to training therapists or in offering treatments to the public. This philosophy seems to be, as data shows, an important aspect of how this sector works and one of the reasons given as to why stakeholders who participated in this study reported they would continue to persist in their work, even in a hostile environment. Another theme to emerge from the data which had not been expected was the reported persistence of this community to continue its work in the provision of training which provides therapists much in demand, as demonstrated earlier in this study for this sector. Many of the learning provider stakeholder experiences should have been enough to make them give up attempts at academic validation, which when rejected, leaves them without recognition and validation of their training programs, and their students and graduates without acknowledgement and recognition of their learning. The education, training and regulator stakeholders who participated in this study report they will continue to persist in their efforts to achieve a framework of recognition for this community, and those whom they represent.

In exploring this community of learning providers, professional regulators and practitioners across the diversity of CAM therapies, the focus of this study was to examine the concerns and needs of this sector, within both the quantitative and qualitative elements of this study. The following questionnaire results demonstrate that most CAM stakeholders surveyed report that the lack of any form of recognition for the sector, and the lack of national registration of therapists is a key concern. Academic validation of CAM training courses and recognition of their qualifications goes hand in hand with recognition of the sector, and was a continuous thread of concern throughout this study. Alongside their main concerns are the needs of this community which are demonstrated in the following chart and document Recognition of their sector, National Registration of therapists, and Academic Validation and Recognition of their training programmes as being core needs for this community.

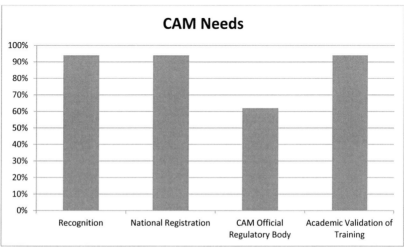

Figure 6.1: CAM Needs from Q3 Questionnaire

All of these results are supported by the text box comments and qualitative interviews in which the majority of respondents cited recognition of all aspects of CAM training and practice as being a key need for this community. All CAM stakeholders, without exception believe there should be acknowledgement and recognition of the work that they do, and recognition of the training that they undertake. There is a stated acknowledgement within this community, that this sector is different to the main biomedical healthcare sector, however, the experience of CAM therapists is that they provide a valuable therapeutic healthcare choice for those who actively seek their expertise and services. Study data confirms that respondents believe this should be acknowledged and recognised within its own context.

These are some of the following of the comments from some of the most experienced and most active respondents in relation to the needs of the sector. It was felt that their words reflected best what data collected in this study demonstrated what the Irish CAM community needs are.

"It is vital for public safety to have qualifications validated and to have practitioners registered so that they adhere to agreed code of practice and ethics" Respondent 4, Q 3.

A practitioner who also has the role of a regulator made the following comment.

"I'd like to see the government be a bit more proactive about our position, there doesn't seem to be a place for us within healthcare setup I was just speaking to the chair of the Dutch XX Association and he was telling me that in their government, they have a very different role. Here we are unique in that we are not regulated here we are in some sort of a niche. We are delivering a good service, which is beneficial and we are regulated and registered in other states within the EU, but not here. There should be a provision to recognise us and regulate us and that should be the same for most of the CAM therapies. I would like to see the government engage more with the sector. The therapies that have a lot of research that showed good effects like Osteopathy, Chiropractic, Acupuncture, Chinese medicine, and give us the opportunity to present our case, I would like to see some session of Parliament deal with this to protect our title, recognise us" Interview No 10 Ireland.

A comment from the following respondent who is a practitioner and regulator suggests a CAM council as one solution.

"One of the National Working Group recommendations was the setting up of the Council, which is the CAM council…. how

178

I would envisage it as a CAM Council is one which would have and develop programs that would be appropriate for all of us, and to contain common aspects of training at code of practice which we all use" Interview No 6 Ireland.

6.1.1 CAM in the UK Comparison

CAM stakeholder data collected from UK, EU and other international participants, within the quantitative and qualitative elements of this study, demonstrate similar issues of concern and need, as outlined from the Irish CAM stakeholders. While the absence of academic validation is not a concern for UK CAM stakeholders, recognition of their professional status and identification of a place within the UK healthcare structures, as part of a formal regulatory framework has been identified by them as a primary need for their communities.

The following comment is one from a respondent who had worked for regulation of a CAM therapy both in the UK and in Ireland.

"I want statutory regulation both in the UK, and I worked very hard for that in the UK, and here as well" Interview No 2, Ireland

There is also, according to UK respondent reports a growing climate of vocal anti CAM voices which are a threat to any small concessions this sector has reportedly worked hard to achieve. According to respondents the UK this is a targeted attack on CAM within higher education and the possibility of a regulatory framework. One of the most active UK respondents made the following comment.

"Resistance to recognition of complementary medicine in the UK has never been so high before. I mentioned before BBC have a program at nine o clock, a whole hour attacking homeopathy. Making jokes, laughing, and the last two weeks we have another 2/3 series talking about some ridiculous complimentary medicine like crystal therapy , they're

179

constantly trying to find the bad examples to attack the whole complimentary medicine. It never happened on BBC before, it's gone into the general broader media and now we know the BBC goes to most of the general public" Interview 4 (UK).

As a comparison to the status of this community in Ireland, the CAM community in the UK have made several advances, not yet seen in Ireland. They have, as discussed achieved academic validation and recognition of the qualifications for CAM training, this gives some public access to some CAM therapies both within NHS funded hospitals and within general practise fund holding centres. There has historically been a good working relationship between UK and Irish professional sectors in many CAM therapies, as there is cooperation and information sharing between both sectors. Government initiatives in both countries have been similar through the Lords Report (2000) in the UK and the DOHC (2005) Report in Ireland, Resistance to CAM recognition in Ireland is more subtle than in the UK, but nevertheless it exists. The regulation gap is open for exploitation to those who do not want to see CAM regulated or recognised. This is an area which could be further explored within the UK CAM communities, and with reference to CAM policy makers in the UK.

Advances in public access to CAM and Academic validation of training is not replicated internationally, as respondents from the EU who participated in this study reported there is no public access to CAM therapies in Holland or Spain which is typical of public access to complementary therapies within the EU. In Brazil a distinction is made between medical personnel who offer some CAM therapies, and non-medical personnel who offer CAM therapies. Non-medical learning providers provide community clinics which offer low cost treatments to the public for some therapies, and there is limited public access to CAM therapies when provided by medical personnel. The UK is not alone in vocal anti CAM campaigns and new voices are emerging in Australia, whose CAM sector have already achieved federal government recognition for a limited number of therapies. That is replicated within the EU and the US as previously indicated in an earlier chapter.

6.2 Conclusion

This research sought to answer the questions which underpinned this study, so that the current status, concerns and needs of this community could be identified and would emerge from the data. Firstly, it was necessary to identify who the CAM stakeholders were, and what their role and representation of their community was. The study explored this community using a mixed methods approach, already discussed, from the historical context of this sector in Ireland, through to their current status and implications of this status. It explored whether their lack of acknowledgement, recognition and regulation has an impact on this community and whether this limits or restricts their work in terms of training and practice, and access to the public. It canvassed the direct opinions and experiences of active representative stakeholders in this community, in terms of history, experiences, issues or concerns across the sector. It canvassed their opinions and points of view on what their community needs so that they may continue their work and find their place within a broad health or therapeutic sector in Ireland. Finally, it identified the needs of this community which emerged from both the quantitative and qualitative data derived from this study, and present the Irish CAM community model as typical of the sector in countries across the world.

6.3 Recommendations.

This study has demonstrated that there have been government initiatives which conducted dialogue and consultation within the broader CAM community in an effort to facilitate a framework of regulation for a broad spectrum of complementary therapists. This initiative in Ireland resulted in the Report on the Regulation of Complementary Therapists, which explored and dealt with the complexity of the whole sector, categorising therapies in terms of risk, treatment and service to the public. It made several recommendations, including one of statutory regulation for some complementary therapies, which had been identified within the report as category one therapists in terms of risk to public, and it recommended a continuation of voluntary self-regulation for other therapies. DOHC (2005 Pg. 45) Similar international government initiatives resulted in the Lords Report in the UK, and parallel EU sector consultative initiatives, none of which resulted in government action or change of status for the CAM sector. What has emerged from this study is that those CAM stakeholders active within their communities need and would welcome facilitation of a framework of recognition and regulation from their governments.

6.3.1 1st Recommendation

A Regulatory Framework for the regulation of this sector should be facilitated by government.

A strong element which emerged from both datasets in study is that the professional structures should be supported, and facilitated by government oversight in the design of a framework of regulation, or the inclusion of CAM in an existing framework of legislation for health and social care workers. The template for this framework already exists in Ireland within CORU the Health and Social Care Professional Council, established in 2010 by government with the role of a multi profession health regulator. Similar legislative structures exist in the UK, and within EU countries to permit inclusion of this sector within the allied healthcare sectors.

6.3.2 2nd Recommendation

Government should re-engage with and facilitate the CAM voluntary self-regulatory structures and their work within the CAM community, as their own report recommends. DOHC (2005)

The recommendation which emerged from the qualitative element of this study is that government should re-engage with   CAM communities with a view to facilitating their inclusion within this existing framework of regulation. Professional associations, who have voluntarily regulated the sector   should be supported and guided towards achieving the *"robust"* self-regulation both Irish and UK government reports refer to, Ibid.

6.3.3 3rd Recommendation

Lifting of suspension of academic validation of CAM programmes

Academic validation of CAM courses at all levels in the national framework of awards should be restored. There is no rationale for a continuation of this suspension and the removal of the awards standards for complementary therapies by HETAC/QQI. Ireland as an active member of the OECD, and the EU, have a role to play in terms of equity and inclusion, routes of access and acknowledgement of lifelong learning, for their citizens. This emerged from the qualitative data and was supported by the literature in this study. Government acknowledgement and accreditation of all learning should be included within OECD and EU member country educational strategies, so that all adult learning has a route to academic validation, within their own communities.

6.3.4 4th Recommendation

CAM community should work together to press for government action in their sector

Leaders and policymakers within the CAM community should engage with each other with the goal of encouraging government action on a variation of the recommendations of the National Working Group Report (2005) and the subsequent SMCI report (2012). EU, OECD, UNESCO should be consulted in this effort to press government for equality and inclusion for this community. This could be used as a strategy for all OECD and EU member countries.

6.3.5 5th Recommendation

Public Access to CAM treatments should be available

This study has demonstrated there is not only a demand for CAM therapies, but there is good evidence of benefits and effects. CAM treatments are currently limited to those who can pay for them, and there is a large population who could benefit from treatments but who have no access to them. CAM treatments with good evidential backgrounds should have a role in both preventative medicine and in occupational healthcare. This would not only make treatments available to those who could benefit from treatments for long term illness, but has the potential to save money on healthcare budgets, and relieve some pressure on hospital and GP services. The use of CAM could support healthcare services in all countries with CAM expertise and availability.

This study has demonstrated that it did examine, identify and present an analysis and an illustration of the needs of CAM communities, as articulated by the representative stakeholders from Ireland, the UK and the many countries whose representatives took part in the research, which formed the basis of this publication.

6.4 Limitations of this study

This study explored the needs of CAM communities, focusing on Ireland as an example of a first world country with a history of natural healing, and traditional governmental conservatism. Ireland is typical of many other first world countries who are members of the OECD and the EU .and have committed their governments to their ideals and those of UNESCO and the United Nations, but who fail to act on those ideals. The CAM sector all over the world has had very little direct research carried out within the context of their own communities, many of the studies carried out have been from the outside, looking in. . I would have liked to further explore obstacles to recognition and the rationale for the reported resistance from some sectors to recognition and formal regulation of CAM therapies, in Ireland and in other countries with similar communities. The study also touched on the different philosophies of life and work, some respondents referred to in their interviews, and as this was spoken about passionately by some of the respondents, this is an area which could be explored further, both in terms of practitioner treatment and therapeutic result. I would like to, at some point, conduct a further exploration of this sector, as either of these areas could benefit from further research, which may further inform national and international CAM communities and those members who sustain their activities..

References

Adami, M.F. and Kiger, A.(2005) The Use of Triangulation for Completeness Purposes.[Online] Available from: http://www.ncbi.nlm.nih.gov/pubmed/16045044[Accessed 8th June 2013]

AONTAS (2014) , *History and Development of AONTAS* [Online] Available from: http://www.aontas.com/about/whoweare/history.html..[Accessed 10th May 2014].

Bodeker, G. Ong, C. Grundy, Burford, G. & Shein, K. (2005) *WHO Global Atlas on Traditional, Complementary and Alternative Medicine.*[Online];. Available from: http://apps.who.int/iris/handle/10665/43108 Pg. 10 [Accessed 2nd September 2013]

Brown, K.L, (2014) *Needs Assessment Report for IERI Research Centre* [Online] Available from: http://drdc.uchicago.edu/eval-activs/needs-assessment-rpt.pdf; [Accessed 5th April 2014]

Bryman, A. (2007). Barriers to Integrating Quantitative and Qualitative Research. *Journal of mixed methods research*, 1(1), pp 8-22.,

Bryman, A. (2014) Triangulation [Online] Available from:
http://www.referenceworld.com/sage/socialscience/triangulation.pdf
pp1-4[Accessed 10th May 2014]

Budd S & Mills S (2000), *Regulation in Complementary and Alternative* Medicine, British Medical Journal.[Online] Available from:
http://www.ncbi.nlm.nih.gov/pmc/articles/PMC1119419/ Pg.
8[Accessed 4th Oct 2013]

CAMbrella,(2012), *The Roadmap to CAM European Research, An explanation of the CAMbrella project and its key findings*[Online]
Available from:
http://www.cambrella.eu/aduploads/cambrellaroadmap.pdf Pg.
2,10,15, 23. [Accessed 5th March 2013]

CAMbrella (2012) *Press Release.*[Online]. Available from:
http://www.cambrella.eu/aduploads/cambrellaroadmap.pdf Pg.
10,[Accessed 5th March 2013]

Cardoso, S, Carvalho, T. Santiago, R. (2011) .From Students to
Consumers: *"reflections on the marketisation of Portuguese higher education" European Journal of Education*, London,
Blackwell.[Online] Available from: http://dx.doi.org/10.1111/j.1465-3435.2010.01447.x [Accessed 7th May 13th 2012]

Cavanagh ,S. & Chadwick, K.(2005).*Health Needs Assessment A Practical Guide*; UK NICE National Institute of Health and Care
Excellence.[Online] Available from:
http://www.nice.org.uk/media/150/35/Health_Needs_Assessment_A
_Practical_Guide.pdf. [Accessed April 2014]

Chandola A, Young, Y, McAllister J, & Axford J S, (1999). *Use of Complementary Therapies by Patients Attending Musculoskeletal Clinics*. London Journal of the Royal Society of Medicine. [Online] Available from http://www.ncbi.nlm.nih.gov/pmc/articles/PMC1297030/[Accessed June 2014]

Collins, J. & Porras, J.(1994) Built to Last Successful Habits of Visionary Companies, US, Harper Business.

Collins, J. (2001), Good to Great Why Some Companies Make the Leap and Others Don't US, Harper Collins.

Colquhoun. (2008). Regulating Quack Medicine Makes Me Feel Sick. *The Times*.[Online] Available from: http://www.timesonline.co.uk/tol/comment/columnists/guest_contribu tors/article4628938.ece[Accessed 6th June 2011]

CORU,(2014) *Health and Social Care Professionals Council*,[Online] Available from: http://www.coru.ie/ [Accessed December 2013]

Creswell, J.(2003) Research Methods, Quantitative, Qualitative and Mixed Methods Approach, 2ndEdition.[Online] Available from: http://isites.harvard.edu/fs/docs/icb.topic1334586.files/2003_Creswe ll_A%20Framework%20for%20Design.pdf [Accessed 6th May 2014]

Creswell, J. W. (2007). Concerns Voiced About Mixed Methods Research. Paper presented at the International Qualitative Inquiry Congress, University of Illinois.

Dawson, C (2009) Introduction to Research Methods, A practical guide for anyone undertaking a research project. Oxford, UK, Howtobooks, Pg. 14.

Denscombe, M. (2010). The Good Research Guide For Small-scale Social Research Projects. 4th ed. Pp 35, 137,138,182,241.Berkshire, UK, Open University Press.

Denzin, N. (2006). Sociological Methods: A Sourcebook.. US, Aldine Transaction. (5th ed.)

Department of Education and Science (2000), *Learning for Life, White Paper on Adult Education.* Dublin: Stationary Office.

Dillman, D. A. (2000). Mail and Internet Surveys: The Tailored Design Method (Vol. 2). New York: Wiley

DOHC ,(2001).*Quality and Fairness, A Health System for You.* [Online] Available from: http://www.dohc.ie/publications/pdf/strategy.pdf?direct=1 Pg. 122. [Accessed May 2014]

DOHC(2005)National Working Group for the Regulation of Complementary Therapists[Online] Available from:http://www.dohc.ie/publications/complementary_therapists.html ,Pg.s5,7,11,16,22,32{Acced on [5th February 2013]

Elliott, R., Fischer, C. T. & Rennie, D. L. (1999). Evolving guidelines for publication of qualitative research studies in psychology and related fields. *Br. J. Clin. Psychol.* 38(3): 215–229.

EACEA,(2009). Adults in Formal Education: Policies and Practice [Online] Available from: http://eacea.ec.europa.eu/education/eurydice/documents/thematic_r eports/128EN.pdf[Accessed 10th February 2014]

ECOTEC, (2007). *European Inventory on Validation of informal and non-formal learning.* [pdf] [Online] Available from: //www.ecotec.com/europeaninventory/publications/inventory/Europe anInventory.pdf. [Accessed December 2011].

Ernst , E.& White, A. (2000) *"The BBC survey of complementary medicine use in the UK" Complementary Therapies in Medicine.*[Online] Available from: http://linkinghub.elsevier.com/retrieve/pii/S0965229900908331 Issue 1, March 2000 Pp 32-36 [Accessed 2nd Feb 2013]

EUROCAM, (2012). *European Public Health Alliance (EPHA).*[Online] Available from: http://epha.org/IMG/pdf/Press_Release_Complementary_Alternative _Medicine_Conference.pdf [Accessed 5th January 2-13]

Europa,(2014). Directive 2004/24/EC of the European Parliament and of the Council of 31 March 2004 . [Online] Available from; http://eur-lex.europa.eu/legal content/EN/ALL/;ELX_SESSIONID=TrKGTypRdnMlQchyvNz5JrJ1Y FWXW09ppjLDhtPVsJFCW2QL6vn0!- 1781699526?uri=CELEX:32004L0024. [Accessed 8th November 2013]

Europa, European Commission, (2006) *Communication from the Commission. Adult learning: It is never too late to learn* [Online] Available from:. http://europa.eu/legislation_summaries/education_training_youth/life long_learning/c11097_en.htm [Accessed 5th December 2013]

Europa, European Commission, (2007). Communication of the Commission to the Council, the European Parliament, the European Economic and Social Committee, the Committee of the Regions – Action Plan on Adult Learning: It is always a good time to learn.[Online] Available from: http://www.eesc.europa.eu/?i=portal.en.soc-opinions.19149 [Accessed 6th December 2013]

Europa, (2009).*Education and Training 2020 (ET 2020), Council Conclusions on a Strategic Framework for European Cooperation in Education.*[Online] Available from: http://europa.eu/legislation_summaries/education_training_youth/ge neral_framework/ef0016_en.htm. [Accessed 15th November 2013].

Europa, (2011) *Adults in Formal Education. Policies and Practice in Europe. Education, Audio visual and Culture Executive Agency.*[Online] Available from: http://eacea.ec.europa.eu/education/eurydice/documents/thematic_r eports/128EN.pdf[Accessed 10th February 2014]

Fenech Adami, M.F. & Kiger, A. (2005), *Nurse Researcher 12.4 19-29* [Online] Available from: http://www.ncbi.nlm.nih.gov/pubmed/15607250 [Accessed 10th September 2013]

Fitzsimons, P. (2002) *Neoliberalism and education: the autonomous chooser Radical Pedagogy (2002) ISSN: 1524-6345 ISR Issue 71, May–June 2010* [Online] Available from; http://radicalpedagogy.icaap.org/content/issue4_2/04_fitzsimons.ht ml [Accessed 21st May 2012]

Glesne, C. & Peskin, A. (1992) Becoming Qualitative Researchers, An Introduction, London, UK, Longman, Pg. 104.

Glaser, B. G & Strauss A.L (1967), The Discovery of Grounded Theory Strategies for Grounded Theory. California US Adline Transaction.

Gibson, W. and Brown, A. (2009) Working With Qualitative Data, London, UK, Sage Publications, Pg. 197.

Green, J.C.(2007), Mixed Methods in Social Enquiry, San Francisco, US, John Wiley & Sons,. Pp 7, 20, 98, 143,144,181.

Guerin, S.& Hennessy, E. (2002). Pupils definitions of bullying, *European Journal of Psychology in Education. Vole XVII, No3, 249-261.*UCD, Dublin.

Hart, C,(2008), Doing a Literature Review, Oxford, Sage. Pg. 26

HEA (1998) *1998 Amendments to the Higher Education Act of 1965*[Online] Available from http://www2.ed.gov/policy/highered/leg/hea98/index.html. [Accessed on 3rd September 2013]Pg. 11

HETAC, (2011).*Update on the Validation of programmes in complementary therapies.*[Online] Available from: http://www.hetac.ie/docs/May%2012th%202011%20Combined%20 web%20notice.pdf [Accessed 8th June 2012]

HETAC, (2012) .*Guidelines and Criteria for Quality Assurance Procedures (2011)* [Online] Available from;http://www.hetac.ie/docs/H.2.4- 2.0_Guidelines_and_Criteria_for_QA_Procedures.pdf [Accessed 13th May 2012]

HETAC, (2010). *Standards for Complementary Therapies* [Online] Available from: http://www.hetac.ie/docs/CT%20Standards%20Sept08.pdf [Accessed 4th March 2014]Pg. 1.

Horner, W. Dobert, H. Von Kopp, B, Mitter, W (eds) 2007,*The Education Systems of Europe.* Netherlands, Springer Science and Business Media.

House of Lords (2013),*Science and Technology – sixth report* [Online] Available from: http://www.parliament.the-stationery-office.co.uk/pa/ld199900/ldselect/ldsctech/123/12301.htm [Accessed 15th March 2013]

Johnson, R.B. & Onwuegbuzie, A (2004) *Mixed Methods Research. A Research Paradigm whose time ha*s come[Online] Available from: http://edr.sagepub.com/content/33/7/14.short [Accessed 15th March 2013]
193

Katz-Haas, R. (1998). *User-centered design and web development.* [Online] Available from: http://www.stcsig.org/usability/topics/articles/ucd%20_web_devel.ht ml [Accessed 15th February 2014]

Kennedy ,J .F. (1963). *Civil Rights Speech,*[Online] Available from: http://www.milestonedocuments.com/documents/view/john-f-kennedys-civil-rights-address/text [Accessed 10th February 2014]

Mc Donagh, S. Devine ,P. & Baxter, D.(2007) *Complementary and alternative medicine, patterns of use in Northern Ireland. Research Update,* [Online] Available from: http://pure.qub.ac.uk/portal/en/publications/complementary-and-alternative-medicine-patterns-of-use-in-northern-ireland%28b90c57e6-c12d-4ca7-9033-ea5cdb2930fb%29.html [Accessed 12th December 2013]

Mc Donald ,S .K .& Parks, K. (2003), Needs Assessment Report for IERI Scale Up Research Projects.

McKillip, J., Bickman, L. & Rog, D (eds) 1997. *Need analysis: Process and techniques. In Handbook of applied research methods* (pp. 261-284). Newbury Park, CA: Sage.

Mc Namara, G.O Hara, J.O Sullivan (2008) *Contexts and Constraints An Analysis of the Evolution of Evaluation in Ireland with Particular Reference to the School Sector*[Online] Available from: http://www.dcu.ie/education_studies/cee/documents/contexts_and_c onstraints.pdf [Accessed 10th September 2013]

194

Maguire, M .(2004), An Introduction to Complementary Medicine *Therapeutic Scope – Complementary Therapies*, [Online] Available from: https://www.icgp.ie/assets/56/85C6ED46.../1-4%20Complementary.[Accessed May 2014]

Mason J (2006)

Real Life Methods Six strategies for mixing methods and linking data in social science research, [Online] Available from: http://eprints.ncrm.ac.uk/482/1/0406_six%2520strategies%2520for%2520mixing%2520methods.pdf Pg. 3. [Accessed 10th March 2014]

Mathison, S (1988) *Why Triangulate. /educational researcher*, 17(2), 13-17.[Online] Available from: Mathison, S (1988) Why Triangulate. /educational researcher, 17(2), 13-17. [Accessed on 20th February 2-14]

Mays, N. & Pope, C.(eds) 2000,. Quality in qualitative health research Qualitative Research in Health Care (2nd edition). London: BMJ Books. pp. 89-10

Medlin C, (1999) *World Wide Web Versus Mail Surveys; A comparison and Report*.[Online] Available from: http://anzmac.org/conference/1999/Site/M/Medlin.pdf [Accessed 20th September 2013]

Miles, M..B. and Huberman ,A .M .(1994) Qualitative Data Analysis, 2nd Ed, Oxford, UK, Sage, Pg..42

Miles, M..B. Huberman, A. M .and Saldana, J.(2014) Qualitative Data Analysis A Methods Sourcebook 3rd ed.
195

Miles (2008) Happy Twaddle Free Birthday to the NHS2. *The Times* [Online]. Available from:http://www.timesonline.co.uk/tol/comment/columnists/alice_mil es/article4159652.ece [Accessed 10thJune 2013]

OECD (2003). *Beyond Rhetoric: Adult Learning Policies and Practices.*[Online] Available from: http://www.oecd.org/education/innovation-education/18466358.pdf Pg. 33 [Accessed 12th February 2014]

OECD, 2008. *Education at a Glance – OECD Indicators*[Online] Available from: http://www.oecd.org/education/skills-beyond-school/41284038.pdf [Accessed15th February 2014]

OECD, 2005. *Promoting Adult Learning.* [Online] Available from: http://www.oecd.org/education/innovation-education/35268366.pdf [Accessed 15th February 2014]

O Sullivan, T. (2002) *Report on the Regulation of Complementary and Alternative Medicine in Ireland.*.[Online] Available from: http://www.dohc.ie/publications/regulation_of_practitioners_of_comp lementary_and_alternative_medicine.html, Pg. 1, [Accessed 1oth August 2013]

Patton, M. (1990). Qualitative evaluation and research methods (Pg. 169-186),196.London, Sage.

Peters, D. (2013) *Implementation Research, What it is and how to do it*:[Online] Available from: at http://www.bmj.com/content/347/bmj.f6753: [Accessed 12th February 2014]

Peters T & Waterman R(1982) In Search of Excellence, Lessons from Americas Best Run Companies, Australia, Harper & Row.

Phillips (2004) St Brigid [Online] Available from http://www.catholicculture.org/culture/liturgicalyear/activities/view.cf m?id=1289 [Accessed November 5th 2013]

Polit D.F.& Beck C.T (2010) Generalization in quantitative and qualitative research: Myths and strategies *International Nursing Student* .Vol 47, 11, 1451-1458, Elsevier B.V, England

Pope, C. Zibland, S. and Mays, N. (2000), Qualitative research in health care. Analysing qualitative data. BMJ Jan 8;320 (7227):114-6

Punch K, (2010) Introduction to Social Research, Quantitative and Qualitative Approaches, London, Sage, Pg. 235

Quality and Qualifications Ireland (2014) *National Framework of Qualifications*.[Online] Available from http://www.qqi.ie/Pages/National%20Framework%20of%20Qualifica tions.aspx [Accessed 8th January 2014]

Ravitch, S .& Riggan, M. (2012),*Reason & Rigor, How Conceptual Frameworks Guide Research*.[Online] Available from http://www.edrev.info/reviews/rev1267.pdf [Accessed 3rd March 2013].

Reviere, R., Berkowitz, S., Carter, C.C., Gergusan, C.G. (eds) 1996. Needs Assessment: A Creative and Practical Guide for Social Scientists. Washington, DC Taylor and Francis:

Ribbins, P & Marland, M. (1994) Headship Matters, Conversations with seven secondary school headteachers, Essex, UK, Longman.

Robson, C .(2002), Real World Research, 2nd Ed Oxford, UK, Blackwell Publishing, Pp 5, 81, 232, 270, 399

Rouda, R. & Kusy, M. (1995), *Needs Assessment, The First Step.* [Online] Available from: http://alumnus.caltech.edu/~rouda/T2_NA.html [Accessed 20th February 2014]

Russom G, *Obama's neoliberal agenda for education* [Online] Available from: http://www.isreview.org/issues/71/feat-neoliberaleducation.shtml. [Accessed on 21st May 2012]

Saldana, J. (2013) The Coding Manual for Qualitative Researchers, London, UK, Sage. Pg., 13, Pg. 239.

Sarsina, R. (2007), *The Social Demand for a Medicine Focused on the Person: The Contribution from CAM to Health and Health genesis* [Online] Available from: http://www.ncbi.nlm.nih.gov/pmc/articles/PMC2206228/Pg. 70. [Accessed 10th April 2014].

Sharples, F. M. C., Van Haselen, R., & Fisher, P. (2003). *NHS patients' perspective on complementary medicine: a survey. Complementary therapies in Medicine, 11*(4), 243-248.[Online] Available from: http://www.ncbi.nlm.nih.gov/pubmed/15022657_ [Accessed 6th June 2014]

Sheehan, K. B. & McMillan, S. J. (1999). Response variation in e-mail surveys: An exploration. *Journal of advertising research*, 39(4), 45-54.

Silverman D (2011) Qualitative Research, 3rd Edition, London, UK, Sage Publications, Pg. 133.

Skillsnet ; *Training Needs Analysis (TNA) Guide*. [Online] Available from: http://www.skillnets.ie/sites/skillnets.ie/files/imce/u7/tna_guide_2013. pdf [Accessed on 10th April 2014]

SMCI (2012) *Review on the Academic Validation of Complementary Therapy Programmes*. [Online] Available from: http://www.dohc.ie/press/releases/2012/20120905.html?lang=en Pg.s1 – 3, ,Pg. 7, 8, 37 [Accessed 10th October 2013]

Strauss. A.& Corbin, J.(1998), *Basics of Qualitative Research. Techniques*[Online] Available from: https://researchandeducation.wikispaces.com/file/view/Open+Codin g.pdf Pg. 274, [Accessed 10th January 2014]

Susanti, D. (2011). *Privatisation and marketisation of higher education in Indonesia: the challenge for equal access and academic values.*[Online] Available from: http://link.springer.com/article/10.1007/s10734-010-9333-7#page-1 [Accessed 25th June 2013]

Survey Monkey Website www.surveymonkey.com

Thomas, K. J.& Nicholl, J. P. & Coleman, P.(1998) *Use of Complementary Use of complementary or alternative medicine in a general population in Great Britain.*[Online] Available from: http://www.ncbi.nlm.nih.gov/pubmed/11264963, Pg. 156. [Accessed 10th January 2013]

Tsutsui, W. M. (1996)   Deming and the Origins of Quality Control in Japan [Online] Available from: URL:http://www.jstor.org/stable/132975 [Accessed 15th May 2012

Titcomb A.L.(2000), *Needs Analysis, ICYF Concept Evaluation Sheet.*[Online] Available from:http://extension.arizona.edu/evaluation/sites/extension.arizona.edu.evaluation/files/docs/needs.pdf [Accessed April 2014]

Tyler, R. W. (1949). Basic principles of curriculum and instruction. Chicago: US University of Chicago Press.

UNESCO (2014) *Education Development Goals.*[Online] Available from: http://www.unesco.org/new/en/education/themes/strengthening-education-systems/quality-framework/development-goals/ [Accessed 20th April 2014].

200

UNESCO (2014) *General Education System Quality Analysis/Diagnosis Framework GEQAF)*[Online] Available from http://www.unesco.org/new/en/education/themes/strengthening-education-systems/quality-framework/Pg.s 6,17. [Accessed 20th April 2014]

US Gov Admin; (2001) *Comprehensive Needs Assessment; Office of Migrant /education New Directors Orientation*; [Online] Available from: http://www2.ed.gov/admins/lead/account/compneedsassessment.pd f_ [Accessed 10th April 2014]

Van Selm, M., & Jankowski, N. W. (2006).*Conducting online of Quality and Quantity,*[Online] Available from: [Accessed http://link.springer.com/article/10.1007%2Fs11135-005-8081-8#page-1 [Accessed August 2013]

Vasquez A (2006) *AMA Declares War on Naturopathic Medicine, Patient Safety and Freedom of Choice in Health Care.* [Online] Available from: http://www.naturopathydigest.com/archives/2006/aug/editor.php Pg. 2_ [Accessed February 2014]

Walker & Budd. (2002) *The Current State Of Regulation Of Complementary And Alternative Medicine.* *Complementary Therapies in Medicine,*[Online] Available from: http://linkinghub.elsevier.com/retrieve/pii/S0965229902905224[Acce ssed [Accessed 12th Mar 2013]

Ward (2009) The Absence of Regulation for Acupuncture and Traditional Chinese Medicine in the UK and Ireland affects the clinical relationship.UK Middlesex University. Department of Social Sciences, Pp 15, 54, 65,68, 71, 78.

Walliman, N.(2008) *Your Research Project*, London, Sage, Pp 12,14,16

Watt, J. (1997). Using the internet for Quantitative Survey Research. Quirk's Marketing

Research Review [Online] Available from: http://www.websm.org/db/12/1217/Web%20Survey%20Bibliography/ Using_the_Internet_for_quantitative_survey_research/ [Accessed 3rd December 2013]

Webb, E. J., Campbell, D. T., Schwartz, R. D., and Sechrest, L. (1966). *Unobtrusive Measures: Nonreactive Measures in the Social Sciences.* Chicago: US, Rand McNally.

Werquin, P .(2009) *Lifelong Learning in Europe 3.*[Online] Available from: http://www.oecd.org/education/skills-beyond-school/41851819.pdf Pp 144,145 [Accessed 3rd March 2014]

White, A. R. Resch, A. L.& Ernst, E. (1997) Complementary medicine: use and attitudes among GPs UK. [Online] Available from: http://fampra.oxfordjournals.org/cgi/content/abstract/14/4/302 [Accessed 3rd June 2013]

Williams, M. (2000) *Interpretivism and generalisation*, [Online]
Available from:
http://ils.indiana.edu/faculty/hrosenba/www/Research/methods/willia
ms_generalization.pdf [Accessed 15th April 2014]

Wiese A, Kellner, J. Britta, L. Waldemar, T. Zielke, S. (2012)
Sustainability in Retailing – A Summative Content Analysis.[Online]
Available from:
http://www.emeraldinsight.com/journals.htm?articleid=17021623
[Accessed April 2013]

WHO (2000) *General Guidelines for Methodologies on Research
and Evaluation of Traditional Medicine.*[Online] Available from:
http://whqlibdoc.who.int/hq/2000/WHO_EDM_TRM_2000.1.pdf?ua=
1 Pg. 1 [Accessed on 10th November 2013]

WHO (2003), *Fact Sheet No. 134: Traditional Medicine,*[Online]
Available from:
http://www.who.int/mediacentre/factsheets/2003/fs134/en/.
[Accessed 20th September 2013]

APPENDIX A: Sample of Analysis of Question Responses From Q2 Questionnaire. (1)

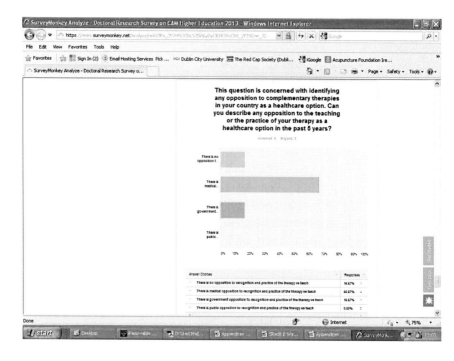

APPENDIX B: Sample of Analysis of Question Responses From Q1 Questionnaire (2)

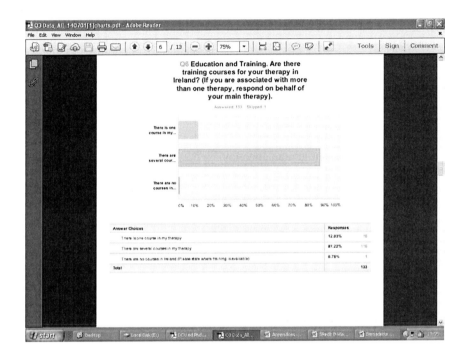

APPENDIX C: Sample of Interview with Irish Learning Provider (Coded)

Code Identification Key:

Role	Recognition & Status	Evidence of Effect	Public Awareness & Demand	Professional Regulation	Employment	Concerns and Needs

HB Interview

B . What is your therapy?

H I run a 4 year course in Western herbalism, I am the course director at my partner is the course coordinator.

B. How long have you been doing this?:

H we started the course in 2000. I suppose that's 14 years now.

B is it a private institution.?

H. Yes, it is a completely private institution it privately funded. We received about XXX a few years ago. From there, X Y Y. to help us with the garden herb garden equipment, computers and setting up the website and web design. Part of the course, but it's completely funded by ourselves.

B . Going back to when you first started, how did you prepare your course?

H. Initially I was running a very busy practice. I wanted to retire and not retire and cut back a little, but I also felt I had a responsibility to teach people about herbal medicine in Ireland, just as I had been taught as I thought this would die out .

Even in England a similar school in herbal medicine, shut down and it had shut down because I think there was a lot of talk about regulation. I think learning providers were a little nervous about regulation so that seem to be the reason why it shut down so there was a sense of having to keep that alive here, so initially, what did I do. I suppose initially, I ran the course is the same model as the course. I studied in England and I spoke to a couple of colleagues in England who would have had some experience in education and medical herbalist and I negotiated with them to come over and take some classes or 8 to 12 weekends a year.

I hired facilities in Maynooth, University. It was a weekend heavy course and we started teaching and then at the end of the first year we had one teacher and then we had another it became quite like laborious for groups, all running at the same time in four rooms in Maynooth South campus.

Material was all delivered in the days with printing it was before the Internet, There was a lot of photocopying and the printer invariably broke down and I think of it, there was two or three printers constantly going to provide people with notes, but that's how we did it, but it soon became apparent, that we needed clinical training and we started that in this small clinic in Dublin. Then it became very laborious because students would have to attend all these weekends and also attend the clinic's. Clinical training became our biggest challenge, but we provided it with great cost to or energy and finances, because it's very difficult to run the student clinic. As you know, because you have to take care of your patients. You have to take your students. They have to feel they are being educated, you have to pay all the costs you have to pay all your staff and you have to make that cost-effective. That is when the whole thing about training started all of this was self-funded would have gotten bank loans ourselves, but we funded it all ourselves from student fees.

B . Why did you feel you have to do clinical training was this big asked a few or did you realise it yourself.

H . No, I realised it. I suppose I knew because I had such a lack of it in my own education in the early 80s I had a good academic education, but no clinical or practical, but I felt that what I could bring to the teaching was many years of clinical experience because I had worked for years as their herbalist, says the age of

24 or 25 right up until my late 30s and I felt I had a lot of experience to date, but with that at that time I was starting to look at models of best practice is an various things and we came across EHTPA a bad day had a curriculum with a certain number of clinical hours and this was the accepted as a standard , but it became apparent to me that this is what we would have to do on both levels and that this is what would be required for regulation.

B . So did you benchmark your course against the EHTPA standard?

H. Initially, when we put our course together, we used the EHTPA, a curriculum as a model as far as they recommended number of hours for each part of the course was concerned. For example, pathology, a certain number of hours theory, a certain number of hours clinics a certain number of hours, so we did it that way. Benchmarking is, I suppose what you would call it.

Then we had an interesting experience. We were invited by an Institute of technology, a rural institute to Institute in fact, and we were invited in fact, courted by them to run a course and together with their but that didn't work out, but during the process. I started to get a sense of the HETAC requirements. The course material that needed to be presented and how you write an academic modules so that was a learning experience, so I suppose now, of course, is benchmarked against the EHTPA model but also against the BSC honours level of HETAC or QQI.as they are known now. As you know HETAC never went ahead with validation of complementary medicine at its all been suspended, so it's neither here nor there. But we subsequently had another experience with another Institute, who were very involved as wanted us to have our course and we spent many hours with them and with their people, many hours mapping the course, according to HETAC guidelines , but in the end we pulled away from that. But we did receive a lot of education from that, we learned how to put course plans together..

B. So do you think that it would benefit the course If you linked up with an Institute, which was already an accredited body?

H. Yes we did. We thought if we linked up with them that it would make the course more recognised make the students want to study more on our course make it more acceptable and it would just help the course all round, and there would be a course in Ireland. That would be a degree course and would have some sort of validation from HETAC. During the process. It has got to a very late stage because we had got contracts ready to sign with the Institute from a solicitor and in the end we didn't sign and the reason we didn't sign was because in our many conversations with them. It became apparent that their paradigms with very different to ours and they would have had a nursing school attached, and it would have been a medical model and allopathic medical model theory mechanistic very, very different to natural medicine, which is very vitalistic and holistic and had a completely different philosophical approach them what they wanted to do so.

We felt that the two couldn't go together. Plus, we took a look at what had happened in England and it seemed from my observation is that the private colleges or courses got swallowed up by universities or institutes and of course when you hand over your course to win Institute for and It's up to them whether they run it in year three or year for they tend to make these decisions based on student numbers, so if you have one bad intake, they could stop the course and he would have lost your course. We decided in the end it was not the right direction for us. We valued our independence and we valued our ability to be able to run our own cause holistically and put our own stamp on it, and to preserve our course in herbal medicine training survive as we felt it should

B . Do you use the native tradition in herbalism?

H. We use Irish herbs as much as possible, we use substitutes when we can find them lot of our products come from Europe from Germany from German herbalists from French herbalists and may influence is from a doctor ,

Dr X Y , an American herbalist he would have been trained who lived in the last century and died in the 80s. He was an influential medical herbalist in the European tradition, he would have trained under Sxxxxx one of the experts. They would use diets and is lifestyle as well and the assessment for that would-be iridology Iris diagnosis, so it's that kind of thing in our part of herbal medicine.

It would be very important for us that our students would know how to grow herbs that they would use and that they would learn how to make their own remedies and are really important aspects and one which I am concerned about is in future regulation is their ability to dispense herbs themselves to their patients. Not just to prescribe, but to dispense. I know in Germany. The German herbalists don't dispense. They just prescribe .

A herbalist is a craftsperson and needs to be able to make their remedies themselves at the touch and feel and taste the herbs they prescribe and dispense and to know and to have intuitive bond with their herbs as a craft, just as a baker bakes so every herbalists gives up the right to dispense the are no longer herbalists, so that would be one of my fears about the future of regulation that we might lose that. Regulation can be good for a lot of reasons for good practice safety etc, but if it threatens our ability to practice what herbalists have been practising for hundreds and thousands of years that the problem.

B . D. You think regulation would threaten the ancient crafts or skills?

H . Yes, I think it might it depends on the contrary, and who's doing the regulating of course if the herbalists were involved, then it might be preserved. You have to have hygiene facilities. All of the facilities that practitioners would be happy to answer all of the rules.

APPENDIX D: Sample of Interview with R Head of TCM School in Brazil

May 2013 Penascola, Spain

Role	Recognition & Status	Evidence of Effect	Public Awareness & Demand	Professional Regulation	Employment	Concerns and Needs

B: So I just wanted to talk about higher education and CAM therapies in Brazil, so what is the status of education?

R: Nowadays there is no regulation on any of these in Brazil, official regulation. So what we have is what we call open or free places, which means there is no barrier to accreditation with our Ministry of Education. For Acupuncture and some of the others if you are already a health professional with a reputation for example you can take Acupuncture for two years with an official post-graduation certificate. This certificate is accredited by our Minister for Education, so we don't offer the full Bachelor program but if you have a Bachelor in any kind of health you can take the post graduate certification.

B You mention others, there is Naturopathy graduation in two Universities in Brazil, there are also two Universities offering degrees in Chiropractic?

R   As there is no regulation if you want you can just study Acupuncture, and become an Acupuncturist. But if you already have a Bachelor degree you can take the same program as a post-graduation program.

B: Ok and how runs these programs are they private colleges or..?

R: Most of them private colleges or schools. There are some programs for medical doctors that are offered inside public Universities, but most of them as they are post-graduation they are charged.

B: So what happens then if a non-medical student does the course and completes and gets a certificate, is he/she allowed to practice?

R: Everyone can practise in Brazil as there is no regulation. It is in our constitution that you cannot force someone to do or not do something if there is no law.

B: So it's almost like common law in the UK?

R: It would be similar but it's like a basic component of our constitution. There must be a law to forbid you to do something.

B: And what about the public, do they look for Acupuncture treatments, chiropractic, and osteopathy?

R More and more, there was a study that said there was a growth of about 400%

B: How was the study carried out, was it a survey?

R In Brazil the public health system is always free, so they keep track of everything that they do. So they compared how many people got acupuncture five years ago and last year.

B: So does that mean CAM treatments are included in the public healthcare system?

R I think five years ago there was a new resolution that allowed alternative medicine to be in our healthcare system, but mostly it is acupuncture, and not just practiced by Western doctors, other types of healthcare professional can practice.

B: Is there any research going on in Acupuncture and complementary medicine?

R : Yes, many, many researchers.

B: And where are these, are they privately funded or in the universities?

R : Most of them are in the Universities, as part of the program most students have to do one   piece of small research.

B: Like a pilot study is it?

R: It could be pilot study, it could be different it depends on the student. Our own school tries to give money to the student so the research is a good one.

B: So can you tell me about your school, how long have you been

R: My school is the Brazilian school of Chinese medicine; we have been going since 2001. Nowadays we have about 350/400 students but the programs are separate in Brazil so two years just for Acupuncture includes 500 hours of clinical practice. Besides that if the student wants they can go for herbs, Chinese Tui Na, and so on.

B: So when they already have the two years they can specialise? How do you provide the clinical practice, do you have clinics?

R: My own school has a clinic, the general ambulatory which has 15 beds and the specific ambulatory where we provide cosmetic acupuncture and so on. We are one of the only schools in Brazil that offers treatment every day. And in Brazil my patient pays about 30/35euros a month, this is what we do in order to give back to the community.

B: How do you finance this?

R: This is something I decided to basically do pro bono, and it is also a strategy to ensure more people know about acupuncture. If one guy goes he will tell it to the other and so on.

B: Your school does it have academic validation as a Bachelor's degree?

R: In Brazil there is no such thing; we have academic validation for our post-graduation program?

B: Is there a possibility or a governmental plan to have academic validation for an Undergraduate program for private Universities?

R Even in governmental colleges there is no degree. What we are doing now, we are fighting for a regulation law, and under that law we could have a Bachelor program.

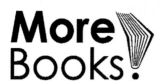
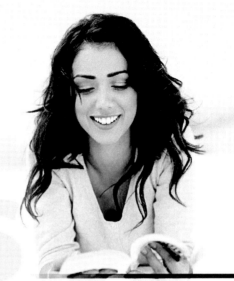

Printed by
Schaltungsdienst Lange o.H.G., Berlin